How to Eat Well When You Have Cancer

Jane Freeman is a highly regarded dietitian and nutritionist with 20 years' experience, whose focus is on helping people undergoing, or who have undergone, cancer treatment. She has been a senior cancer/clinical dietitian within a number of leading Australian public hospitals, a nutrition research manager and product manager with well-known food manufacturers in Australia, and has also lectured in oncology. Jane has worked with the World Cancer Research Fund UK (WCRF), a cancer charity that specializes in cancer prevention research and public health interventions. She wrote the WCRF's publication *Eating Well and Being Active Following Cancer Treatment*. More recently, Jane has been a consultant in Australia and the UK. She is often asked to provide comments in the media, and she has appeared on BBC *Breakfast* and other news programmes.

Overcoming Common Problems Series

Selected titles

A full list of titles is available from Sheldon Press,
36 Causton Street, London SW1P 4ST and on our website at
www.sheldonpress.co.uk

101 Questions to Ask Your Doctor
Dr Tom Smith

Asperger Syndrome in Adults
Dr Ruth Searle

The Assertiveness Handbook
Mary Hartley

Assertiveness: Step by step
Dr Windy Dryden and Daniel Constantinou

Backache: What you need to know
Dr David Delvin

Birth Over 35
Sheila Kitzinger

Body Language: What you need to know
David Cohen

Bulimia, Binge-eating and their Treatment
Professor J. Hubert Lacey, Dr Bryony Bamford
and Amy Brown

The Cancer Survivor's Handbook
Dr Terry Priestman

The Chronic Pain Diet Book
Neville Shone

Cider Vinegar
Margaret Hills

Coeliac Disease: What you need to know
Alex Gazzola

Coping Successfully with Pain
Neville Shone

Coping Successfully with Prostate Cancer
Dr Tom Smith

Coping Successfully with Shyness
Margaret Oakes, Professor Robert Bor
and Dr Carina Eriksen

Coping Successfully with Ulcerative Colitis
Peter Cartwright

Coping Successfully with Varicose Veins
Christine Craggs-Hinton

Coping Successfully with Your Hiatus Hernia
Dr Tom Smith

Coping Successfully with Your Irritable Bowel
Rosemary Nicol

Coping When Your Child Has Cerebral Palsy
Jill Eckersley

Coping with Anaemia
Dr Tom Smith

Coping with Asthma in Adults
Mark Greener

Coping with Birth Trauma and Postnatal Depression
Lucy Jolin

Coping with Bowel Cancer
Dr Tom Smith

Coping with Bronchitis and Emphysema
Dr Tom Smith

Coping with Candida
Shirley Trickett

Coping with Chemotherapy
Dr Terry Priestman

Coping with Chronic Fatigue
Trudie Chalder

Coping with Coeliac Disease
Karen Brody

Coping with Diverticulitis
Peter Cartwright

Coping with Drug Problems in the Family
Lucy Jolin

Coping with Dyspraxia
Jill Eckersley

Coping with Early-onset Dementia
Jill Eckersley

Coping with Eating Disorders and Body Image
Christine Craggs-Hinton

Coping with Envy
Dr Windy Dryden

Coping with Gout
Christine Craggs-Hinton

Coping with Headaches and Migraine
Alison Frith

Coping with Heartburn and Reflux
Dr Tom Smith

Coping with Life after Stroke
Dr Mareeni Raymond

Coping with Life's Challenges: Moving on from adversity
Dr Windy Dryden

Overcoming Common Problems Series

Coping with Manipulation: When others blame you for their feelings
Dr Windy Dryden

Coping with Obsessive Compulsive Disorder
Professor Kevin Gournay, Rachel Piper and Professor Paul Rogers

Coping with Phobias and Panic
Professor Kevin Gournay

Coping with PMS
Dr Farah Ahmed and Dr Emma Cordle

Coping with Polycystic Ovary Syndrome
Christine Craggs-Hinton

Coping with the Psychological Effects of Cancer
Professor Robert Bor, Dr Carina Eriksen and Ceilidh Stapelkamp

Coping with Radiotherapy
Dr Terry Priestman

Coping with Rheumatism and Arthritis
Dr Keith Souter

Coping with Snoring and Sleep Apnoea
Jill Eckersley

Coping with Stomach Ulcers
Dr Tom Smith

Coping with Suicide
Maggie Helen

Coping with Type 2 Diabetes
Susan Elliot-Wright

Depressive Illness: The curse of the strong
Dr Tim Cantopher

Divorce and Separation: A legal guide for all couples
Dr Mary Welstead

Dying for a Drink
Dr Tim Cantopher

Dynamic Breathing: How to manage your asthma
Dinah Bradley and Tania Clifton-Smith

Epilepsy: Complementary and alternative treatments
Dr Sallie Baxendale

The Fertility Handbook
Dr Philippa Kaye

The Fibromyalgia Healing Diet
Christine Craggs-Hinton

Free Yourself from Depression
Colin and Margaret Sutherland

A Guide to Anger Management
Mary Hartley

The Heart Attack Survival Guide
Mark Greener

Helping Children Cope with Anxiety
Jill Eckersley

Helping Children Cope with Grief
Rosemary Wells

High-risk Body Size: Take control of your weight
Dr Funké Baffour

How to Beat Worry and Stress
Dr David Delvin

How to Cope with Difficult People
Alan Houel and Christian Godefroy

How to Develop Inner Strength
Dr Windy Dryden

How to Live with a Control Freak
Barbara Baker

How to Lower Your Blood Pressure: And keep it down
Christine Craggs-Hinton

How to Manage Chronic Fatigue
Christine Craggs-Hinton

Hysterectomy: Is it right for you?
Janet Wright

The IBS Healing Plan
Theresa Cheung

Let's Stay Together: A guide to lasting relationships
Jane Butterworth

Living with Angina
Dr Tom Smith

Living with Asperger Syndrome
Dr Joan Gomez

Living with Autism
Fiona Marshall

Living with Bipolar Disorder
Dr Neel Burton

Living with Crohn's Disease
Dr Joan Gomez

Living with Eczema
Jill Eckersley

Living with Fibromyalgia
Christine Craggs-Hinton

Living with Gluten Intolerance
Jane Feinmann

Living with IBS
Nuno Ferreira and David T. Gillanders

Living with Loss and Grief
Julia Tugendhat

Living with Osteoarthritis
Dr Patricia Gilbert

Living with Osteoporosis
Dr Joan Gomez

Living with Physical Disability and Amputation
Dr Keren Fisher

Overcoming Common Problems Series

**Living with a Problem Drinker:
Your survival guide**
Rolande Anderson

Living with Rheumatoid Arthritis
Philippa Pigache

Living with Schizophrenia
Dr Neel Burton and Dr Phil Davison

Living with a Seriously Ill Child
Dr Jan Aldridge

Living with a Stoma
Professor Craig A. White

Living with Tinnitus and Hyperacusis
Dr Laurence McKenna, Dr David Baguley
and Dr Don McFerran

Losing a Child
Linda Hurcombe

Losing a Parent
Fiona Marshall

**Making Sense of Trauma: How to tell
your story**
Dr Nigel C. Hunt and Dr Sue McHale

Menopause in Perspective
Philippa Pigache

Motor Neurone Disease: A family affair
Dr David Oliver

The Multiple Sclerosis Diet Book
Tessa Buckley

Natural Treatments for Arthritis
Christine Craggs-Hinton

Osteoporosis: Prevent and treat
Dr Tom Smith

Overcome Your Fear of Flying
Professor Robert Bor, Dr Carina Eriksen
and Margaret Oakes

Overcoming Agoraphobia
Melissa Murphy

Overcoming Anorexia
Professor J. Hubert Lacey, Christine Craggs-Hinton
and Kate Robinson

Overcoming Emotional Abuse
Susan Elliot-Wright

**Overcoming Gambling: A guide for problem
and compulsive gamblers**
Philip Mawer

Overcoming Hurt
Dr Windy Dryden

Overcoming Jealousy
Dr Windy Dryden

Overcoming Loneliness
Alice Muir

**Overcoming Panic and Related Anxiety
Disorders**
Margaret Hawkins

Overcoming Procrastination
Dr Windy Dryden

Overcoming Shyness and Social Anxiety
Dr Ruth Searle

Overcoming Tiredness and Exhaustion
Fiona Marshall

**The Pain Management Handbook:
Your personal guide**
Neville Shone

Reducing Your Risk of Dementia
Dr Tom Smith

**Self-discipline: How to get it
and how to keep it**
Dr Windy Dryden

The Self-Esteem Journal
Alison Waines

Sinusitis: Steps to healing
Dr Paul Carson

Stammering: Advice for all ages
Renée Byrne and Louise Wright

Stress-related Illness
Dr Tim Cantopher

Ten Steps to Positive Living
Dr Windy Dryden

**Therapy for Beginners: How to get the best
out of counselling**
Professor Robert Bor, Sheila Gill and Anne Stokes

Think Your Way to Happiness
Dr Windy Dryden and Jack Gordon

**Tranquillizers and Antidepressants: When to
take them, how to stop**
Professor Malcolm Lader

**Transforming Eight Deadly Emotions
into Healthy Ones**
Dr Windy Dryden

The Traveller's Good Health Guide
Dr Ted Lankester

Treating Arthritis Diet Book
Margaret Hills

Treating Arthritis: The drug-free way
Margaret Hills and Christine Horner

Treating Arthritis: More ways to a drug-free life
Margaret Hills

Treating Arthritis: The supplements guide
Julia Davies

Understanding Obsessions and Compulsions
Dr Frank Tallis

Understanding Traumatic Stress
Dr Nigel Hunt and Dr Sue McHale

The User's Guide to the Male Body
Jim Pollard

When Someone You Love Has Dementia
Susan Elliot-Wright

Overcoming Common Problems

How to Eat Well When You Have Cancer

JANE FREEMAN

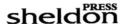

First published in Great Britain in 2012

Sheldon Press
36 Causton Street
London SW1P 4ST
www.sheldonpress.co.uk

British Library Cataloguing-in-Publication Data
A catalogue record for this book is available from the British Library

ISBN 978-1-84709-141-3
eBook ISBN 978-1-84709-280-9

Typeset by Fakenham Prepress Solutions, Fakenham, Norfolk NR21 8NN
Printed in Great Britain by Ashford Colour Press
Subsequently digitally printed

eBook by Fakenham Prepress Solutions, Fakenham, Norfolk NR21 8NN

Produced on paper from sustainable forests

Contents

List of illustrations   viii

Foreword by Dr Michelle Kohn   ix

Foreword by Dr Clare Shaw   xi

Introduction   1

1   Nutrition in cancer   7

2   The impact of cancer and its treatment on the body   15

3   Monitoring your nutritional health in cancer   27

4   Cancer treatments: what to expect and how to prepare   34

5   Preparing for treatment at home: ways to eat well (with
    recipes)   43

6   Coping with side effects: nausea and vomiting, taste
    changes and fatigue   72

7   Coping with side effects: others (pre- and post-surgery,
    constipation, diarrhoea, etc.)   89

8   Food safety and preventing infections   118

9   Common questions   124

10 After treatment: a word on healthy eating and cancer
    prevention   133

Conclusion   142

Appendix: Drink and meal supplements   146

Useful addresses   151

Further reading   155

Index   157

Illustrations

Figures

3.1	Body Mass Index (BMI) chart	33
5.1	The Eatwell Plate	57
5.2	The 'high-protein' Eatwell Plate	57
5.3	The 'build-up' Eatwell Plate	58

Tables

3.1	Nutritional risks associated with different types of cancer	28
4.1	Common nutritional side effects of radiotherapy	40
5.1	Fast- and slow-release carbohydrates	45
5.2	Foods providing approximately 10 g of protein from both higher and lower quality types of protein	49
5.3	ORAC antioxidant capacity of selected fruits, vegetables, grains and legumes	65
5.4	Herbs and spices	69
6.1	Getting through a day when you feel nauseous	78
7.1	Tips for soft foods	98
7.2	Build-up trolley v. weight-management trolley	115
10.1	Some simple ideas for bringing more phytonutrients into your day	140
A.1	Nutritional supplement range	146

Foreword

DR MICHELLE KOHN

When you are diagnosed with cancer, it can be genuinely hard to work out what and how to eat. You are bombarded with dietary advice and confronted with alarmist and confusing media stories, but given very little concrete information by the busy doctors who treat you.

As a doctor specializing in integrative cancer care, and the emerging field of cancer survivorship, I have long had an interest in cancer and nutrition. I am the director of Living Well, a non-profit programme based at the cancer treatment centre, Leaders in Oncology Care. Living Well guides patients through the emotional and practical minefield of cancer treatment and beyond. We were lucky enough to have Jane working with us for two years to devise a nutritional programme for patients and their carers and I am thrilled that she has turned this expertise into a book.

There is strong medical evidence that eating well can make a real difference to how patients cope with cancer treatment and its side effects. Good nutrition, combined with exercise, will not only improve your quality of life and help you manage your symptoms, but it may help to stave off a recurrence of cancer. And yet many patients just don't know where to start with all this. I see many who have adopted wacky, stressful and unwise regimes, perhaps excluding whole food groups, in an attempt to 'beat the odds'. Others, meanwhile, just throw up their hands and ask, 'What's the point?'

Cancer treatment can have a major impact on how and what you eat. It can bring weight gain or weight loss and side effects such as nausea and fatigue, as well as appetite, digestive or taste changes. When life already seems out of control, this can seem like the last straw. That is where Jane comes in.

Jane fully understands the medical side of cancer. She is not just rigorous and scientific, though, she is sympathetic and practical; she understands that food should be healthy, but also enticing, easy to prepare and delicious. Food should not take over your life, but it should certainly enhance it.

Jane understands that no two people have the same nutritional, personal or medical needs. She offers tips, here, for meeting whatever your specific challenges are, from taste changes to fatigue or digestive issues. She demystifies common questions such as the value of supplements, or the soya debate in hormone-sensitive cancers. And she explains how to eat for overall future health, rehabilitation, and to prevent recurrence. This is all rooted in the growing body of scientific evidence. But above all, it is do-able.

During her workshops at Living Well, Jane would often include pictures of herself in her kitchen at home, cooking with her children. She understands the reality of food shopping, preparation, cooking, and eating for pleasure. She offers an astonishing combination of kitchen table wisdom (focusing on the kind of fresh, wholesome food that grandma would have made) and cutting-edge nutritional research. She isn't dogmatic and doesn't lay down strict rules, because she understands real life.

At Living Well, people often said to me, after Jane's workshops, 'If only I'd known this from the start . . . but my oncologist said just eat what you like.' So much distress could be avoided if cancer patients and their carers could see Jane as soon as they were diagnosed. She has already helped hundreds through her work as a specialist oncology dietitian, and through Living Well – and will continue to do so, since she is so generously donating the profits of this book to us. And now you, too, can share her wisdom and expertise in your own kitchen at home.

This book is an invaluable resource. It will help you to enjoy food again and to feel confident and nourished, and I am delighted to recommend it.

Dr Michelle Kohn MB BS BSc FRCP
Director
Living Well Programme
Leaders in Oncology Care (LOC)

Foreword

DR CLARE SHAW

One in four people will be diagnosed with cancer in the Western world. There are also millions of people living 'with and beyond' their cancer diagnosis as treatments for cancer have improved significantly in the past few decades.

Being diagnosed with cancer is the beginning of a physical and emotional rollercoaster for the person and their family and carers. There are many challenges along the way, and eating and drinking a good healthy diet is certainly one of them. We are constantly bombarded by the stories in the media relating to food and our health and it can be difficult to decide on the best advice to follow. Good nutrition underpins health and is essential to support the body during rigorous cancer treatment; but achieving the right balance, and maintaining it, can be a huge challenge.

Food impacts enormously on our daily life. Eating is a social occasion; it brings together family and friends and is essential to sustain life. But illness, particularly cancer, can profoundly affect our food intake. In a short period of time turmoil around food preparation and eating may occur – leaving the person with cancer and their carers struggling to keep the right balance.

It is not uncommon for people to lose weight prior to their diagnosis; in fact this may be one of the early symptoms that alert us to the fact that something is wrong. This may easily get overlooked as the process of diagnosis and treatment planning gets under way but it may remain a constant source of worry. People may question whether their diet has contributed to their cancer, be too afraid to eat or may just struggle because the cancer is affecting their appetite, taste and enjoyment of food.

The nature of cancer treatment may make eating even more difficult. A succession or combination of treatments – surgery, chemotherapy, radiotherapy and endocrine therapies – can influence appetite and food intake in many ways. Symptoms from cancer and treatment combine to create a hostile environment for eating well. Taste changes, poor appetite and nausea are just some examples of symptoms that people may experience, suddenly making an enjoyable daily activity something to be dreaded or avoided.

Working with people with cancer for many years has taught me that the best ideas come from those who are struggling and have found what works for them. In *How to Eat Well When You Have Cancer* those ideas have been brought together with the scientific evidence underpinning good nutrition. This book will help guide people during those difficult times, when thinking of what to eat is overwhelming. At a time when many aspects of life are out of control, it is important to be able to manage this vital part of everyday life. Practical advice to inspire and tempt people is invaluable, particularly when it is based on sound nutritional knowledge. This book also recognizes the emotional component of eating – of preparing food for another person, of nurturing them to withstand the rigours of cancer as a disease and its treatment.

Hopefully this book will provide invaluable support to both the person with cancer and their carer, to ensure that eating remains one of life's great pleasures.

Dr Clare Shaw
Consultant Dietitian
The Royal Marsden NHS Foundation Trust

Introduction

The other day at work, I was taken by surprise by the daughter of a lovely lady whom I had seen some years ago. She came up to me and said, 'Aren't you the nutritionist who got my mother through? Do you remember how you helped her to get her strength back and gave her the energy to get through her treatments?'

While of course I remembered the daughter, with whom I had been in close contact, it was her mother who took me by surprise. Sitting in the waiting room was a radiant lady – smartly dressed, glowing and looking fantastic. This was certainly not the person I had met some years before, whom I had been asked to see quite urgently early on in her treatment.

At the time, I remember she was very frail, her mood and morale were very low, and she had lost her way with food. In addition, she was having specific difficulties absorbing her food because of gut surgery.

I learned that this lady had been an amazing cook and very much the food matriarch of the family. So it was hard for her and her family to cope with the fact that she simply did not want to eat, and certainly cooking was the last thing she could face. We had to spend some time talking through the reasons why good food was so important to her body's nutritional and energy needs at that time, and we also had to explain to her and the family why she did not feel like eating or wanting to take food.

The next stage, working out some reasonable and realistic options, had to be approached carefully, with constant adjustments. The important point that had to be made to the family was that, at times, all the best intentions in the world cannot manufacture a healthy appetite in the person with cancer. Their efforts to prepare the right food and an inviting eating environment were very understandable, but also needed to be balanced by an awareness that these efforts weren't always going to work. In short, they needed to respect the times when their mother really did not want to eat or just couldn't manage it. It can be very hard for families to recognize that pressing a person to eat may imperceptibly turn into nagging. When mealtimes become a food war, it is a horrible situation for all concerned. It is difficult for families to accept that a person with cancer is never refusing food because she does not have the will to go on, but simply because she can't bring herself to eat.

As this lady did not live locally, we continued to stay in touch during the following months by phone, email and regular texts. Although it was not easy, she was able to work her way forward with a mixture of some simple, soft foods that were easy to take, along with some special milkshake drinks that were put together for her. Her daughter also kept a food diary on her behalf, which I was able to review and add to with ideas that might help. While I had heard she had done very well and had finished her last course of chemotherapy treatments at our clinic some time ago, now, when I actually saw her in for a review appointment, I was very struck by the change in her. The sight of her looking so well showed how a combination of medical treatments and nutritional support had brought this lady from a very low point to where she is today.

Engaging with nutrition

Engaging with nutrition is one of the most important aspects of cancer treatment that individuals and their families can become involved in. While cancer and its treatment may have varying outcomes, treatment options are improving and many people are living well with cancer for many years. Making the effort to eat a good diet is therefore vital.

Enjoying foods which support you before, during and after your treatment will help you feel better, stay stronger, tolerate treatment side effects better, keep up your energy, maintain your weight, reduce the risk of infection and heal and recover as quickly as possible.

During the active stage of treatment, you need what I might call an intense nutritional approach. This isn't a matter of fad diets or of cramming yourself with special foods, but of good, sound nutrition. Treatment for cancer affects people in many ways, but thinking about it as a kind of marathon event may help you understand what kind of role you play in your nutrition – an active one, I hope. If you were training for a marathon or planning a long trek up a mountain such as Everest, I am sure you would understand the importance of fuelling your body to help you build up your strength and stamina, and as preparation for recovery from the physical and psychological impacts you were about to endure. You would need to organize yourself with extra rations and supplies in case of problems or unforeseen challenges that might arise on your journey.

Beating cancer is never easy, whether you are in the throes of treatment or simply living with it in the best way you can. In any case, understanding the right way to eat can give you a real boost, help you recover, and give you the extra energy and strength you need to fight on. So, taking an active part in your diet and liaising with a healthcare team who can help provide specific guidance is something that I hope you will welcome.

Many people are only too keen to make changes in their diet but aren't always sure of the best way to go about it. There is a great deal of conflicting advice around and it can all be very confusing. Some people are convinced that certain foods cause cancer, while others advocate very restricted diets in the interests of a 'cure'. As diet is one area where people with cancer can take control, it is understandable that they are sometimes eager to make the most of the opportunity. Equally, if people aren't eating well and find it all too difficult, this can be a source of concern and guilt. What I want to say to you right from the start is: relax and take it easy. A top oncologist once told me that his advice to patients asking about nutrition was to 'eat what you fancy', and while I would add a little detail to it, this kind of spirit is very much what inspires this book. Food is to be enjoyed and to nourish the body. It's not some kind of arcane magic that you must get exactly right if you are going to be cured. So I do ask you to try and put negative preconceived ideas out of your head and read this book with an open mind.

This book will help guide you through the possible side effects of the treatments, together with aspects of the cancer itself that may impact on your appetite and ability to tolerate your normal diet.

Throughout the book I will describe how nutritionists like me, along with other cancer health specialists, are involved in your treatment – and why we want to know how you are doing with your diet, how your weight is tracking and whether you are experiencing any problems, and if so, what we can do to help manage them.

I must say how privileged I am to have worked with many people such as this lady, who have shown an enormous amount of strength and courage in the way they have taken on the nutritional advice provided. I have had so much pleasure from witnessing how good nutrition has given them a sense of involvement and control that other aspects of their medical treatment may take from them.

The essence and purpose of this book

My desire to work with food and nutrition stemmed from the deep influence my mother had on me. Although, sadly, I lost her to cancer early in my career, she left an enormous imprint on me in a love of food and cooking, and this has continually fuelled my passion to pursue these interests. Working with individuals with cancer is a constant source of inspiration and challenge.

I particularly wanted to write this book to share how food and nutrition can help feed your soul, can help you get that bit more out of your day and can give you another source of pleasure, or at least a reason to spend more quality time with friends and loved ones. My mother always served up good food, even when she was not well. I witnessed how important it was for her to still seek out the best quality ingredients, and how much pleasure she got bringing friends and family together at our big dining table with a succulent roast, lots of colours of root vegetables, the best potatoes – and always an amazing pudding to finish off with.

Taking this passion for good food with me, I wanted to help guide people to the nutritional approach or support that would make the most difference during their treatment. Diet in cancer is a highly emotive area and one where there is a great deal of myth and misunderstanding. I want to help you cut through the confusion and the nonsense and false promises. I want you to know when to go for a wholesome green bean salad or when you're much better with Mum's home-made chicken soup, a warming cottage pie, or a poached egg on a piece of buttered toast.

So I will be giving you some information about nutrition and cancer and suggesting ways to approach your diet, with several ideas for overcoming eating difficulties, backed up with recipes of my own as well as from my patient collection. Above all, I want you to understand that eating the right way when you have cancer and beyond should not be particularly complicated. When you can eat normally, it will be all about good food that nourishes you, and all you need can be brought from supermarkets, farm shops, markets or the local fishmonger, butcher and other speciality stores who can tell you more about where the produce is from. It is about simple recipes, it is often about short cuts, it is about freezing meals ready to go and it can be about eating out and savouring good food experiences. This is especially important if it means spending time with friends and family, or easy options if you are tired or need a lift.

It is not about pills, potions or the latest superfoods. It doesn't have to be organic, super-green, filled with extra antioxidants or in line with any other food fads. It is certainly not about feeling miserable, about being restricted or about total avoidance; nor is it about seeking out weird foods or excessive juicing. I want this book to help you connect with good food, balance and taste, and to understand the main role for nutrition, both during your treatments and beyond.

While nutrition has a key role to play in supporting people during their cancer treatment, there are no particular foods or food groups which have been shown to be an absolute cause of cancer. Nor are there any special or restricted diets which have been shown to cure or significantly reduce risks of recurrence. Hence what is most important during treatment for cancer is that you temper a healthy, balanced approach to your diet with a flexibility of approach. This means being prepared to adjust or modify aspects of your diet, adding foods as necessary, so that if you are facing challenges you can try to ensure that you are going to meet all your basic nutritional requirements. This simply means eating in whichever way you need to, so that you try not to lose or gain significant amounts of body weight over the treatment period.

Thus the purpose of this book is simply to give reliable, practical information on the role of nutrition in cancer treatments at the key stages. It covers some crucial nutritional recommendations for people with cancer, to help them cope with the treatments and the side effects. But, most importantly, it suggests an approach that combines the best eating for you with sheer enjoyment of food. It is designed to help you look out for new ideas for sourcing great quality produce, and suggests ways to enjoy your regular recipes, to learn to adjust them if needed, or to try out some of my simple recipes. I hope you will find a way to savour good tastes, to be decadent as often as you can and always to focus on the other reasons for the importance of eating occasions, such as their social significance. Having a ritual such as a regular family evening meal can be a very important anchor during the day, and a chance to relax, connect and exchange information. You're much more likely to enjoy your food in the relaxed context of eating with loved ones. While at times eating can be difficult during treatment for cancer, try not to let these challenges get in the way of spending the time at a table catching up with family and friends and, most important, looking out for lots of special mouthfuls just to treat yourself and your taste buds.

Good nutrition is simply knowing what your priorities are at this moment and knowing what foods agree with you or can best be tolerated. These might be the ones that are easy to digest, the ones you crave, the ones that can give back and that will nourish you and your soul. It is about ensuring you have enough of everything during the day or the week to get you feeling as well as you can, besides giving you the strength to tolerate the treatments advised by your consultant as giving you the best possible chances. It is also about sometimes recognizing the need to be a little novel, inventive and willing to experiment, or being prepared to eat differently from your usual patterns if the going is a little tough. This can be very hard for some people, and I hope this book will be able to guide you and to explain the need for changes in your diet that you might previously have thought of as being unhealthy.

I hope you find my book helpful, nourishing and edible. *Bon appetit.*

Note on recipes

Measures in recipes are based on the Australian standard cup, which holds 250 ml (8.75 fluid oz). A useful chart of metric and imperial equivalents can be found at <www.taste.com.au/how+to/articles/369/weights+measurement+charts>.

1

Nutrition in cancer

When we are well, most of us do not usually spend too much time thinking about the connection between eating and taking in the many food nutrients our body needs daily to keep it all ticking along and functioning well, never mind managing the many extra tasks that take a fair bit of effort and energy, including thinking, breathing, moving, warding off bugs and infections, breaking down the food, converting it into a form the body can use like petrol, rebuilding and repairing cells, getting rid of waste products and so much more!

Most of us also do not really think about how amazing our body is. We may not realize how much work it does each day even before we get out of bed, and we probably won't think about how our food can affect the body's ability to do all it needs to do.

That is, we won't normally think about it until we have to deal with the shock of a diagnosis like cancer, which then quite understandably sends people into a state where they agonize over what they might have eaten or been exposed to in their life. And unless this is quite obvious, they often make nutrition into a kind of quest, exploring diet as a way of trying to explain why they have been struck with cancer. This is especially so when they have lived normal healthy lives or the cancer has presented at an early age.

So while it is true that a poor diet, inactivity and an excessive alcohol intake are key risk factors in around 30 per cent of cancers, it is important to recognize that they are not the only reasons for cancer. Instead of specific dietary causes *per se*, it is more about how good your genetic hardware is, and then your body's ability to deal with both the good and bad environmental exposures in your life experiences.

This is so important, as once you are diagnosed the immediate priority is to work with your medical team to decide which treatments are going to give you the best outcome. This also means looking at which approach to diet will give you the most nourishment and the additional support you need to cope.

If you do not have any food problems, it is certainly reasonable to keep eating a normal healthy protective diet. However, in case of difficulties – if weight loss is a problem, say – then alternative dietary strategies will need to be employed. However, now is not the time to embark on some prudish anti-cancer meal plan which restricts your intake of the foods that give you the most support and nourishment to help boost blood counts, give you energy and help you to cope.

It never ceases to amaze me that someone who is about to start treatment for cancer should think that taking on some sort of extreme or greatly restricted dietary approach will help his or her body to do well. I sometimes explain that in many ways a cancer journey and the treatments should be approached as if you were about to take on a long-distance trek through the mountains or, in some cases, an extreme endurance event like the Tour de France.

There is nothing wrong with wanting to use nutrition to support and protect yourself, but before you write out the shopping list or proclaim the merits of the latest diet book you need to be sure that the approach you have researched is in fact the right one for you.

This can be quite confusing, as unlike many other chronic illnesses such as heart disease or diabetes, where diet approaches are reasonably standard, diet for cancer is quite specific to the type and stage of the cancer.

Cancer is quite a heterogeneous disease, and as its causes centre around the complicated processes the billions of cells in our body go through to divide and replicate every second of the day, it is hard to pin down the causes. There are more than 200 different types of cancer, there are different stages of the disease, and there are many options for and combinations of treatment, which can include surgery, chemotherapy, radiotherapy and biological treatments. In addition to the various effects cancer itself has on the body, the treatments themselves often contribute their own set of challenges and side effects.

It is also important to recognize that everyone with cancer has a different starting point, and simply adopting broad-brush recommendations or a radical internet diet is often not what is needed by your body at this time.

How can good nutrition make a difference?

Doing your best to eat to meet your energy (calorie) and protein requirements during the treatment is so important. When the body is not receiving the nutrition it needs, it is rather like trying to run the car when the petrol tank is empty.

Today I was called in to see a lovely gentleman who informed me that all he had been eating was fruit and 'a few extra bits' over the past few weeks. During this time his weight had dropped a further 10 kg (22 lb) to 59 kg (130 lb). He was having trouble getting up and taking a shower, and he just didn't feel like going out or catching up with friends. He was very weak, and when I left him he immediately fell asleep.

While some of the reasons he was having trouble with his food had to be unravelled with the medical team, the key issue was that, as his food intake was well below ideal, he had become malnourished. His body was so run down that the actions of getting out of bed, sitting in a chair and taking a shower were all a challenge. Little wonder he felt so low in himself, with limited interest in getting out with friends, not to mention his frustration at having his treatments cancelled because his bloods showed that his body had not recovered from his last dose of chemotherapy. Chemotherapy is normally worked out according to a person's weight, and if there is significant weight loss the dose usually has to be reduced, which can affect the potency of the treatment.

Most of us think of malnutrition as only being a problem in countries of the Global South exposed to famine situations. However, it is one of the biggest problems in the NHS. My gripe is that, all too often, people are referred to me when they have already become extremely malnourished and when their treatment is already significantly under way, instead of earlier on, when intervention would have had a better effect and would have helped prevent the associated complications. We hear so much about the problems of obesity in our society, but in actual fact it is the problems of disease-related malnutrition that cost our health system more. While awareness of disease-related malnutrition is being actively promoted in the community and healthcare institutions, a much greater collaborative effort to intervene earlier is still needed. Like this gentleman, people live with low energy and experience more problems with infection, with the result that their treatments are affected – and often because their nutritional health was left to dwindle.

The more you can do to eat well and embrace the type of diet that can best support you, the better your treatment outcomes are likely to be. This also means being proactive if you are having difficulties, and asking for extra help sooner rather than later.

Your diet can influence the appearance of your skin, eyes, stamina, shape, strength, bowel function, immune system and even mood; doing your best to eat the right sort of foods in the proportions you need at that particular time can really make a difference. This means different things for different people depending on the type and stage of cancer you have, but whatever you can do to ensure your diet supports you in the right way is beneficial.

Ways nutrition helps support your treatment for cancer

Good nutrition helps you to

- cope with optimal treatment options and doses;
- recover and heal;
- maintain a healthy body size and shape;
- better manage treatment side effects;
- reduce some risks of recurrence;
- boost immune system function and fight off infection, preventing unnecessary setbacks and hospital stays;
- feel more energized and cope with common problems associated with fatigue;
- ensure your body is equipped with a good store of the key nutrients such as iron, calcium and zinc, along with other vitamins and minerals;
- improve your ability to concentrate and manage daily tasks;
- improve mood;
- possibly reduce recurrence risks, according to emerging evidence.

How do I need to think about nutrition during my treatment?

One of the most difficult concepts for many people with cancer to grasp is that they may need to adopt very different dietary approaches from those they may have been used to, and from those widely promoted as healthy dietary guidelines. These are the well-known guidelines which recommend eating more fruit and vegetables, grains, lean meats, fish and low-fat dairy foods, and limiting fat, sugar and salt in the diet. They have been represented pictorially over the years as pyramids, healthy plates and the like, and I'm sure you're very familiar with them.

However, it is important to realize that you may need to make some changes to what you know as healthy eating. Usually when people are well they have no trouble eating enough food and can manage the extra bulk and fibre provided by a healthy diet. Owing to treatment side effects and the burden of the cancer on the body, though, you may actually need to reverse accepted ideas about healthy eating and to eat in an opposite way to how you may have eaten in the past. You may need to focus on eating more snacks and higher-calorie foods, using extra butter, salt and at times sugar. Quite often I tell people that they may need to start eating like a stereotypical teenager! This can be quite difficult as most of us have our eating habits fairly ingrained. So I often encourage people who are having difficulties to think back to their teenage years and eat as they may have when it was cool to hang out with their friends at McDonald's and the like. While my views and food preferences are now quite different, I well remember begging my parents to take us out for a burger and my old favourite of a caramel sundae!

If you have a cancer which is not associated with any nutritional problems, remember that guarding against muscle loss and nutrition depletion is the biggest priority during treatments, and it may be appropriate for you to start with a dietary approach recommended for people who are well into their cancer treatments.

Dietitians and their role in cancer treatment

The fundamental role of a specialist cancer dietitian or nutritionist (as some practitioners prefer to be called) is to help mitigate the impact cancer and its treatment can have on your nutritional health. This is important as it relates to how well your body copes with the treatment and to your overall ability to cope. It affects your recovery, your energy levels and your ability to resist infections, and it can also impact on other longer-term health outcomes.

To ensure that we are best placed to give sound advice on diet and cancer, cancer dietitians work hard at keeping up with the scientific literature, including constant reviews of the evidence around diet and the many types of cancer. We also participate in continuing education, which includes attending regular updates with other specialist oncology dietitians. We have meetings with the nutritional supplement companies, we work with colleagues to review best practices, and as most of us work in the NHS or have worked in hospitals we have the advantage of being able to continually learn from our other healthcare colleagues, including doctors, nurses and other cancer specialist practitioners.

In our first meetings with people with cancer, we take time to review their individual situations. This includes not just looking at their medical history and blood results, but also understanding their current situation, their social supports and how they are coping. We find it useful to know what type of cancer they have and at what stage, where they are in terms of their treatment, whether there are any struggles or side effects affecting their dietary intake or tolerance, what they are managing to eat and how this measures up to their current requirements.

I personally also like to know what people hope to gain from their treatment and what they feel are the best and most manageable options for them to engage with so that nutrition will make a difference. People work in different ways, but I have found that many of my patients head home from their day at the clinic quite overloaded with information, not to mention 'chemo brain'. Hence I always put together a personalized food plan that they can put on the fridge door. In addition to outlining the key recommendations, I aim to cram in lots of new and refreshing food suggestions for them to try, or at least to refer to at a later stage. Prescribable nutrition supplement drinks or special feeds may also need to be considered.

There are of course many doctors, specialist nurses and health professionals who advise on nutrition, and this is usually a good starting point for advice in a cancer clinic. However, the benefit of seeing the dietitian is that you can seek out the best options for you, tapping into the expertise and practical nutritional know-how we have acquired from working specifically in this area.

There are many people who claim expertise in nutrition, those I like to describe as the fringe-dwellers. While they make big claims, quite often they do not have any real clinical training or experience. These people can often do more damage than good and can be recognized as the ones who claim that nutrition can cure just about anything. I really hate it when I see someone who walks in after meeting an alternative-type quasi-nutritionist, and who has been promised big outcomes if he or she signs up to a particular nutritional therapy approach. In addition to weird diet recommendations, there is the sheer cost of such programmes, and often people will have spent a fortune on large amounts of supplements. One of the doctors who ran the Living Well programme at our clinic told of a lady she once met who was somehow managing to take 126 nutrition type supplements a day! The internet can also be lethal as far as these kinds of nutritional traps are concerned. I always warn people to be very wary about handing over credit card details or buying supplements on the internet without first talking to their doctor, nurse specialist or a dietitian like me about whether the purchase will in fact provide any real benefit.

The final piece of information you should know is that dietitians are the only legally recognized nutrition health professionals in the UK. They are registered by an independent body called the Health and Care Professions Council (HCPC), which regulates health professions in order to protect the public. The HCPC maintains a register of nearly 8,000 dietitians, and if you go to its website, <www.hpc-uk.org/>, you can check whether or not a practitioner is registered.

As I mentioned, when an individual first consults me I spend time reviewing the medical history, the stage and type of the cancer, the prognosis, treatments completed or planned, any nutritional problems or difficulties with eating normally, blood test results, any changes in bowel function, problems swallowing, taste changes, digestive difficulties, difficulties with nausea or vomiting, and activity and general energy levels.

I will be especially interested in whether a person has had any recent shape or body weight changes and, if so, in considering what might be the main contributory factors. It is important to learn what people normally like to do with their diet and what they are managing at this time. I will want to understand how someone approaches the shopping and cooking and whether any help or support is available, especially when the individual may not be feeling well.

When I meet people I am always very pleased to hear that they are interested in nutrition and have looked at ways to improve their eating habits. However, because of the complex nature of cancer, I always recommend that they take the time to discuss their planned dietary approaches with their medical team, and if possible with a specialist dietitian. The right approach helps make the whole cancer experience more manageable, and I would also hope that people enjoy the extra goodness that can be gained from eating well during their treatment.

2

The impact of cancer and its treatment on the body

When considering dietary approaches, it is important to be aware that cancer and its treatments can be broadly divided into certain key stages. It is important to then understand what effects the cancer and treatments are likely to have on the body at each of these stages, and how the diet should be framed around them. The stages of the treatment are often described as being part of the cancer journey. While some journeys can be relatively straightforward, others are filled with twists and turns which may not take you quite where you had hoped to be. It is important to be as prepared as you can for the entire journey, but also to understand that detours are often part of the course and may require different approaches to the diet.

Key stages in cancer and its treatment

While stages are not clear-cut and tend to cross over, key stages may be summarized as follows. This book focuses on Stage 2, the treatment stage.

Stage 1: Prevention
This is the stage before a first cancer develops, and the dietary focus is on how to balance overall intake so as to reduce the risks associated with cancer development.

The World Cancer Research Fund (WCRF) is a wonderful charity dedicated to research and resource development on diet and exercise for cancer prevention. In 2007 this organization, in conjunction with the American Institute for Cancer Research (AICR), produced a landmark report, known as the Expert Report, which presented seven years of research evaluating the data around diet as a contributing factor to cancer and is the most comprehensive report ever produced on the links between lifestyle and cancer risk. The research was undertaken by leading scientists across the globe and is being used to develop strategies and action plans to help people eat better and be more active, with a view to reducing the risks of cancer. The Report looked at the half-million studies of the relationship between cancer and diet and physical activity, screening them down to 22,000, of which a final 7,000 were deemed relevant. Information from these then formed the basis of the recommendations for cancer prevention, drawn up by a panel of world-renowned experts. This was a rigorous and thorough process, and really constitutes the best advice we have to date globally on how to reduce your risk of cancer. While detailed dietary advice on this stage is outside the scope of this book, the main findings are summarized below.

- Maintain a healthy weight. Be as lean as possible without becoming underweight.
- Be physically active for at least 30 minutes every day.
- Avoid energy-dense foods, particularly processed foods that are high in added sugar, low in fibre or high in fat, and sugary drinks.
- Eat more fruit, vegetables and plant foods, including wholegrains (cereals) such as rice, oats, pasta and bread, and pulses such as lentils, chickpeas and beans.
- Limit consumption of red meats (such as beef, pork and lamb) and avoid processed meats.
- Limit salt intake, salty foods and foods processed with salt (sodium).
- Limit alcohol – if consumed at all, alcoholic drinks should be limited to two a day for men and one a day for women.
- Don't use supplements to protect against cancer – get your supplements from foods, not pills. Research suggests that it's better to choose a balanced diet with a variety of foods rather than high-dose nutrient supplements, in order to reduce your risk of cancer.

Meanwhile I would recommend any family members who want more details to go to the UK World Cancer Research Fund website at <http://www.wcrf-uk.org/>.

Stage 2: Treatment

This is the key stage around which this book centres. It should be viewed as a window of opportunity in which your diet priorities can be geared to support and boost you. There is quite a spectrum of dietary approaches, depending on how well you are tolerating your diet. The basic starting point for people who are fortunate in being otherwise well and who are not having any trouble eating or maintaining a healthy weight is a good varied and healthy diet – do visit WCRF's website. There is more on this in Chapter 10.

However, if you are having even a little trouble, have a more advanced cancer or have simply lost your way with food, it is important to experiment with alternative dietary approaches to help meet your biggest nutritional priority at this time, which is to ensure you are as strong as you can be for your treatment. This may at times require you to eat differently, take supplement drinks or in some cases accept other ways of feeding, called enteral or parenteral nutrition support. This is not the time to start redlining key food groups out of your diet.

Energy intakes

Energy intakes need to match up to the energy your body is using for all the tasks required to function well during your treatments. If you do not meet these requirements, your body will need to take stock and start cutting back on these functions. It is rather like a company which has had to make some of its staff redundant and cancel some contracts because it can no longer afford to pay the wages.

A struggling company may be able to go on as normal for a short while, but sooner or later it will need to make some tough decisions to cut costs so that it can continue to survive. The body often has to make these tough decisions if nutritional supplies continue to fall short of its requirements. Cutbacks will normally be in the areas of functions that are not absolutely essential, such as energy for extra activity, energy for a better mood, energy to think straight and energy for the immune system.

Stage 3: Palliative care

The objective of eating at this stage is to encourage individuals to make the effort to eat as well as possible even if they don't feel like it. Being better nourished helps them have more energy and feel like doing more; it also helps prevent problems due to infection or dehydration.

However, this stage can be difficult, and it is important for family and loved ones to respect the fact that eating is not always easy and can at times cause pain. It can be hard for the family to accept that you may not want to eat, and this can cause a great deal of unnecessary stress and friction. Food is something with which many of us express our love, but it is equally important that family know and respect the ground rules, which include acknowledging that you may not always feel like eating or finishing what's on your plate. It is also important that mealtimes should be celebrated as time spent together and need not be about what or how much you eat. This is also important if you are being fed with a feeding tube. While it can be difficult and feel odd, I still encourage people to make the effort to sit down with the family at mealtimes if this has been the normal ritual. There is much more to the family mealtime than just eating – the focus at this time should be on enjoying each other's company, catching up on news, laughing and having an enjoyable mealtime experience.

Stage 4: A new start

Moving on can vary, as some people will be lucky enough to have stayed quite well during their treatment while others will feel very drained and need more time to recover from the side effects. However, although daunting for many people, it can be the best time to undertake an audit of those not-so-perfect habits around diet, activity levels and other key areas of your life, and work out how to move forward. You may wish to refer to my booklet, *Eating Well and Being Active Following Cancer Treatment*. It can be ordered or downloaded free of charge from the WCRF website (<http://www.wcrf-uk.org/PDFs/EatingWellBeingActive.pdf>.)

The impact cancer and treatment can have on your body

We are fortunate these days to have an ever-increasing range of incredibly potent cancer treatments such as chemotherapy, radiotherapy, biological therapies and surgery. However, in the process of destroying cancer cells, many of the body's healthy fast-growing cells can be damaged. These include bone marrow, which is responsible for blood cell production (this one is the key driver behind the blood counts), the hair follicles, the immune system and the core lining of the digestive tract right through from the mouth (taste buds) to the other end of the bowel. It is the damage done to a good number of these high-turnover healthy cells that often has the most impact. This is the reason for many of the physical symptoms people have during treatment, and at times it will also interfere with your ability to eat well.

At the same time, these are the organs or body parts which are more likely to be drained by poor nutrition. This is because they are working overtime to try to repair the damage, and constant nutritional supplies are required to enable them to be replenished.

How cancer treatment affects normal functions

Digestion and gut immunity

The lining of the digestive tract has two major roles. First, it enables the body to absorb nutrients from the food we eat: the process called digestion. You may not know that the digestive tract or the bowel is considered to be an outer part of the body, rather like an arm or a leg. It is like a brick wall that helps keep unwanted visitors out. The gut also acts as a big security guard or barrier that prevents unwanted bacteria or viruses from getting into the bloodstream where they can cause more serious infections.

When the cells lining the gut are damaged by the effects of some treatments, it can be more difficult to taste and properly digest higher-fibre foods, too much lactose (dairy foods) or too many rich foods. This can also impact on how well the gut is able to prevent what is called the translocation of bugs into the bloodstream, especially if food intake is poor over an extended period of time, when the gut wall becomes thinner and more porous.

Blood cells and blood counts – energy and immunity

Red and white blood cells have many important roles in cancer treatment; if your nutritional health suffers, this can reduce the ability of the body to produce enough blood cells to cope with certain treatments.

Specifically, lack of red blood cells (anaemia) reduces the body's capacity to carry oxygen from the lungs around the body, contributing to fatigue and shortness of breath. This also means there is a reduced amount of oxygen circulating in the body, which affects the function of all body cells and tissues.

The white blood cells are the body's soldiers or defence forces against infections and other internal insults. If you have a low count of white blood cells such as neutrophils you will be at a high risk of infection, and this is why you will be started on antibiotics and told to keep out of public places and to eat a low microbial diet. For more about this, see Chapter 8.

Immunity – the ability to fight infections

Around a third of our nutritional intake is used to keep our immune system functioning. One of the main ways in which poor nutrition can affect this is thinning of key barriers such as the skin and the lining of the digestive tract, as mentioned above. Furthermore, it can cause a significant reduction in body proteins and the specific bacteria-fighting cells such as the white blood cells, with the result that we are less able to fight the cancer.

Cell repair and treatment recovery

During cancer treatment, the body is working overtime to try to heal and to rebuild the damage done to healthy tissues and cells. If the body is not well nourished, this healing process can be slow as the extra nutrients needed are in short supply. If you are having chemotherapy and your blood counts do not recover between treatments, then treatment doses may need to be reduced or delayed. This may affect your treatment response.

Evidence shows that people who are well nourished are able to heal and recover faster than those who are nutritionally compromised. Hospital stays are also normally shorter and associated with fewer complications in people who are stronger and well nourished.

Muscle loss and strength

If you are not eating enough to maintain your weight and meet your increased protein requirements, the body takes on a rationing approach to the fuel supplies it is able to access. It is rather like a petrol strike: when limits are placed on the days you can buy fuel and the amounts available, you will not be able to drive as far as you normally would.

Our bodies use up quite a lot of fuel. In particular, the brain uses a staggering amount – around a quarter of the food energy we consume. Fuel is also need for the pumping efforts involved in keeping the heart and lungs functioning, as well as the liver, the kidneys and other major organs. If a fuel shortage threatens, though, the body's management systems start to make tough rationing decisions. Cutbacks will normally take away the energy needed for activities and functions that are not essential for survival. This may include energy for extra activity, energy for a better mood, energy to think straight and energy for the immune system.

The body also needs a constant supply of glucose to enable the brain and other vital organs to keep functioning. If you are not taking in enough food, it must break down muscle and fat stores to top up supplies. As the majority of the body's protein stores are in the form of muscles, this breaking-down process incurs definite losses which affect tone and strength. And as the arms and legs are not the only stores of muscle, muscle stores are also drained from within the heart, lungs, digestive tract and immune system.

Think, for example, of the main role of the heart and lungs: to enable us to breathe in oxygen and then pump it around the body. When muscle is lost from the heart and lungs, these essential processes can also be affected. This means it takes the body much more effort to breathe in and move sufficient oxygen. Getting rid of waste products, including carbon dioxide, is also done more slowly. This can have a big effect on stamina and energy levels.

Psychological impact

The psychological impact of cancer can be enormous. One of the most difficult areas can be the way loss of appetite or a change in shape can affect people's social life and how they feel about themselves. A change in appearance – either losing or gaining a lot of weight – tends to make people feel very self-conscious, and it is a common reaction to want to hide away or to disguise yourself in unflattering clothes. The way you appear to yourself and others can also be a constant reminder of illness. Many people find it very hard to deal with this.

At times, given the nature of the illness, changes of this kind are almost unavoidable. However, I do hope that such reminders help you realize again the importance of keeping track of your nutritional health, and of finding practical ways in which you may limit the impact of cancer and its treatment. As I've said before, this doesn't always have to involve huge changes or a superhuman quest. Investing in the effort to nibble when you are not feeling hungry and adjusting some of the usual ways you eat are small things that you can do for yourself. Such changes may make a big difference in your treatment outcome, and also will give you more confidence, help you maintain energy, boost your concentration and enable you to keep enjoying the life you want. So if you do look in the mirror and feel discouraged, sad or distraught, bear in mind that while this is a natural reaction, there are also ways you can take action to change things.

Cachexia – the wasting syndrome

Cachexia is a wasting syndrome with loss of weight, muscle atrophy, fatigue, weakness and significant loss of appetite in someone who is not actively trying to lose weight. It is also known as anorexia cachexia syndrome.

There are certain cancers which affect the way the body metabolizes the food that is ingested. Up to six out of ten people (60 per cent) with advanced cancer develop some degree of cachexia. It is also why some people find they keep losing weight despite their best efforts to eat as well as they can.

Cachexia (kak-ex-ee-a) comes from the Greek words *kakos*, meaning 'bad', and *hexis*, meaning 'condition'. 'Anorexia' simply means 'loss of appetite' – though, as mentioned, cachexia is more than a simple loss of appetite. It is a very complex problem involving changes in the way your body normally uses protein, carbohydrate and fat.

It isn't usual to develop cachexia in the early stages of cancer. Cachexia in advanced cancer can be very upsetting and can make you feel very weak. It isn't just associated with cancer, though. It is common in the advanced stages of other illnesses such as heart disease, HIV and kidney disease.

Cachexia is more common in people with lung cancer or with cancers anywhere in the digestive system. The main symptoms are:

- severe loss of weight, including loss of fat and muscle mass
- loss of appetite
- feeling sick (nausea)
- feeling full after eating small amounts
- anaemia (low red blood cell count)
- weakness and fatigue.

The processes of cachexia are not fully understood, but it is thought that the cancer releases chemicals into the blood that contribute to the loss of fat and muscle. These chemicals may make your metabolism speed up so that you use up calories faster – a bit like the body putting its foot on the fat and muscle burn accelerator. Because your body is using up energy faster than it is getting it, severe weight loss may result even if you are eating normally. This may also be exacerbated by the side effects of cancer treatment.

Changes that may occur include the following:

- Fat stores are broken down to top up the body's energy needs. They become difficult to re-stock as the fat is broken down more quickly and the rate at which the body stores fat is reduced.
- Protein requirements are met through a process that eats away at vital organs, muscles and the immune system. This has an effect on the weight lost, and on grip strength and functional abilities. There may also be an increased risk of infection.
- Carbohydrate is burnt for energy at a greater rate and some of this is wasted through inefficiencies, which may account for an additional 300 kcal.

It is also because of cachexia, and the changes in the way the body uses the nutrition that you can ingest, that it becomes very difficult to reverse the weight loss associated with cancer. This is why, if you have cancer, the best insurance policy you can take out is a commitment to early and continued nutritional therapy, particularly if you are having difficulties with your food intake. Protecting your muscle and energy stores and the reserves needed to deal with the treatments is one of the prime goals of your treatment that you personally can attend to.

A word on weight gain

Having waved red flags around the need to nourish your body well and to guard against weight loss, I must stress that it is also important to understand that some types of cancers, mostly the hormonal types, are associated with weight and body fat gains.

Although it is important to nourish your body and to eat in the best way you can during treatment, many people are surprised to discover that they are ravenous a lot of the time and crave more sugary foods. The associated weight gain can vary from around 1–2 kg (2–4 lb) up to 10–20 kg (22–44 lb) in extreme cases.

There are many reasons why certain individuals are prone to weight gain, apart from the types of cancer they have. Certain treatments including hormone therapy, at times the earlier onset of menopause, some types of chemotherapy, and medicines such as steroids can cause weight gain. Some treatments can also cause your body to retain water, which makes you feel puffy and gain weight.

Although there are many factors that contribute to the potential for weight gain, there are two basic prongs in the equation:

1 Because of an increase in appetite and, sometimes, changes in food preferences towards more sugary, high-fat foods, people tend to feel hungry and eat more of these higher-calorie foods. The general rule still holds good: you gain weight when you eat more calories than your body needs.
2 Because of fatigue and feelings of lethargy, there are often changes in activity levels. This means you may not be burning as many calories as before, and the lower levels of exercise mean that you tend to put on more fat weight and to lose muscle. This explains some of the changes in body shape and composition that may also occur.

Weight gain, changes in body shape, feeling fatigued and, for some, hair loss can be difficult pills to swallow. The good news is that the treatments will improve your chances of survival, and the odds are now so much better than in years gone by. At the last count, in 2009, there were around two million cancer survivors in the UK. This is around 13 per cent of the population. Doing what you can to eat well, managing the excessive sugar cravings and being as active as you can are not only helpful strategies to keep you well, but can distract you and pull you through the difficult times. A walk in the park, on the beach or even around an interesting farmer-type market will get you out of the house, and more often than not you will feel so much better for making the effort.

Benefits of exercise during treatment

At our clinic we now have an exercise specialist who advises individuals on suitable activities and programmes. Exercise has many benefits during treatment. It can:

- make you feel better;
- help you maintain a healthy weight;
- boost fitness and stamina;
- build muscle;
- reduce the risk of cancer recurrence.

Of course, at times it is not possible to do as much activity as you may like. It is important to listen to your body to be sure you do not overdo things. It is also best to talk to your doctor and specialist team about an appropriate level of activity for you. For some it may seem difficult to walk as far as the front door or further than the front of the house, while others may feel they can manage to continue much as normal. It is an individual equation; however, unless you are feeling very unwell, try not to hibernate on the couch for too long.

Although this is still an emerging area of research, excessive weight gain during treatment may increase risks of other associated longer-term health conditions such as heart disease and diabetes. Evidence also suggests that it is associated with increased recurrence and so with survival rates.

Sometimes weight gain may be associated with endocrine issues such as insulin resistance, contributing to treatment-associated weight gain. If you find you are gaining weight despite your best efforts to eat well and be active, you should talk to your doctor about your concerns, sooner rather than later.

Diet and nutrition after treatment

The need for good nutrition does not end the minute you walk out of the clinic door for the last time. On the contrary, now is the time to be building up your future health with a vengeance. In addition, the effects of some cancer treatments make themselves felt for several weeks afterwards, so you may need to continue implementing the suggestions given for coping with specific treatments in Chapters 6 and 7. I also look at this subject in Chapter 10.

You also need to bear in mind that, after treatment ends, cancer survivors may be at increased risk of recurrence of the cancer, or of the development of a second cancer or other health conditions such as heart disease, type 2 diabetes and osteoporosis. Your follow-up care will monitor this closely, of course, but, to reduce the risk of further disease, doctors generally recommend that people follow common nutritional recommendations, including eating fruits, vegetables and wholegrains. The effect of specific dietary factors on cancer survival rates is not well understood and is actively being studied. According to WCRF, there is growing evidence that physical activity, a healthy weight and a balanced diet may help to prevent cancer recurrence, particularly for breast cancer. Until this is fully proven, WCRF advises following its recommendations for cancer prevention (visit: www.wcrf-uk.org/cancer_prevention/recommendations.php>). My booklet, *Eating Well and Being Active Following Cancer Treatment*, provides some recommendations and practical suggestions to assist you to take all this forward. It can be obtained for free – see page 18.

3

Monitoring your nutritional health in cancer

While your doctors and specialist nurses can give you the treatments to fight the cancer, eating well and keeping an eye on your nutritional health is your responsibility. Many people welcome this as a key area in which they can have some power, after feeling very much disempowered by the illness and treatment.

Your specialist team will routinely weigh you and monitor any weight loss or gain. However, it is up to you to speak up if you feel you have a poor appetite or are losing weight, if you notice that your clothes are feeling loose or you have specific difficulties eating. Alternatively, if you feel you are gaining weight you should draw it to your team's attention. It is also important to speak up if you have noticed any side effects which are affecting your appetite or your ability to eat normally.

Don't be misled by your current weight, even – or especially – if you are secretly relieved to have lost a few pounds. For example, you may feel that you are overweight but you may still be at risk of malnutrition, as I explain below. When tracking weight, it's more important to look out for fluctuations rather than necessarily going by your current weight. That is, it is more important to record any trends in weight changes rather than what you actually weigh now.

Overweight but malnourished

Recording weight fluctuations is especially important if you were overweight when you started your treatment. Although you may feel or look as if you are currently at a healthier weight, it is still possible for your nutritional health to be compromised. This applies even if you are still at a weight that may normally be considered overweight for your height.

Quite often, people who have started treatment at a weight that would normally be considered higher than ideal are at just as much risk of nutrition or malnutrition problems as anyone else. What needs to be monitored is the amount of weight that has been lost overall, or the total percentage body weight lost over the past one to three months.

People who are overweight may still look healthy or as if they are at a normal weight. However, as their weight may have changed significantly during their treatment, the reality may be that they have lost significant amounts of lean muscle weight and the body may be struggling with the consequences of depleted nutrient stores.

In fact, poor nutritional health issues are often overlooked in someone who appears overweight. Remember to look at weight changes in the recent weeks and months, not just the weight you are at present.

Nutritional problems associated with different types of cancer

Another point to bear in mind is that different kinds of cancer carry certain potential nutritional dangers. Table 3.1 provides a guide to some of the nutritional risks associated with some of the main cancer types. However, because of the enormous diversity in cancer types and treatments this can be no more than a general guide, and

Table 3.1 Nutritional risks associated with different types of cancer

Cancer location	Common nutrition problems	Broad nutrition recommendations
Head and neck	Sore mouth Difficulties chewing and swallowing A third of people experience significant weight loss	Eat very soft food Boost energy intakes Aim for extra support feeding
Upper gastrointestinal tract	Sore mouth and throat Difficulties swallowing Reflux Nausea Two-thirds of people experience significant weight loss	Adopt an early build-up diet Boost energy intakes Eat small frequent meals and snacks

Cancer location	Common nutrition problems	Broad nutrition recommendations
Lower gastrointestinal tract	Risk of nutrition problems depends on stage of cancer and treatments Healthy diet benefits	Fibre intakes may need to be adjusted depending on bowel function If no nutrition problems, then a healthy cancer treatment diet is recommended
Gynaecological (endometrial)	Risk of nutrition problems depends on stage of cancer Weight gain risk Bowel function problems	If no nutrition problems then a healthy cancer treatment diet
Breast cancer	Risk of nutrition problems depends on stage of cancer Weight gain risk	If no nutrition problems then a healthy cancer treatment diet
Prostate cancer	Risk of nutrition problems depends on stage of cancer Higher weight gain risk	If no nutrition problems then a healthy cancer treatment diet
Lung cancer	Risk of nutrition problems and weight loss	Eat to manage treatment side effects and boost diet as needed to help maintain a healthy weight
Brain/ neurological tumours	Risk of nutrition problems depends on stage of cancer Higher weight gain risks due to changes in the endocrine system	If no nutrition problems then a healthy cancer treatment diet
Metastatic or advanced cancers of any type	High risk of nutrition problems and treatment side effects	Eat to manage side effects and boost diet with extra nourishing snacks

Source: Adapted from Dr Clare Shaw, *Nutrition and Cancer*, London, Wiley-Blackwell, 2010, Table 9.1.

you should discuss any individual nutritional concerns with your doctor and treatment team.

If you have a type of cancer that is associated with nutritional difficulties or weight loss, then it becomes even more important to try to eat as well as you can. However, as I said, while it's your responsibility to keep an eye on your nutritional health, do please remember you don't have to do it alone. Indeed, you mustn't – that's what your medical care team is there for!

Are you at risk of nutritional problems?

Here is a simple questionnaire referred to as the Malnutrition Screening Tool (MST), used by many cancer centres to help identify those at risk of nutritional problems during treatment. While a higher score doesn't automatically mean you have nutritional problems, it does flag up those in need of a more thorough nutritional assessment by their doctor or the dietitian.

These simple screening questions should be reviewed on a regular basis, especially if you have a cancer that puts you at risk of nutritional problems or you notice weight or shape changes.

Simply answer the questions below and then add up your scores. Remember, it is just a guide; if you are concerned you should discuss your results with your doctor or specialist nurse team. If you are having problems you should ask to be referred to a cancer specialist dietitian.

1 Have you lost weight recently without trying?
   No: score 0.
   Unsure: score 2.
   Yes: answer Question 2.
2 If you answered yes to Question 1, how much weight have you lost?
   1–6 kg (2–13 lb): score 1.
   7–11 kg (14–23 lb): score 2.
   12–16 kg (24–33 lb): score 3.
   More than 16 kg (33 lb): score 4.
   Unsure: score 2.
3 Have you been eating poorly because of a decreased appetite?
   No: score 0.
   Yes: score 1.

Now work out your total weight loss and appetite score.

A score of 0–1 assumes you are eating well and have not noticed any recent weight loss. Continuing and regular reviews with your team or using this questionnaire are recommended.

A score of 2–3 assumes you are having difficulties with your eating and not managing your normal approaches. It also assumes you have lost between 1 and 6 kg (2 and 13 lb). It is important you inform your team of the difficulties you may be having and request a referral to the dietitian as soon as possible.

A *score of 4–5* suggests you have been having a lot of difficulty eating and have lost a large amount of weight, more than 6 kg (13 lb). It is important to contact your doctor and specialist team for immediate guidance and support. (Based on M. Ferguson, S. Capra, J. Bauer and M. Banks, 'Development of a valid and reliable malnutrition screening tool for adult acute hospital patients', *Nutrition* 15, 6 (1999): 458–64.)

If it is difficult to weigh yourself, or you aren't quite sure how much weight you have lost, or when, then you can look for other clues such as:

- changes in where you buckle your belt;
- whether your rings are becoming loose;
- whether you can observe changes in your face;
- whether people have noticed that you may have lost weight;
- whether your eyes look a little more sunken than usual.

If you note any significant changes here, you should record this as a score of 3 or 4.

At times, the scales can be misleading, especially if you are experiencing fluid build-up (oedema or ascites) around the belly, legs or hands. This type of weight gain is not an indication of excess nutrition. In fact, quite often behind the fluid weight gain many individuals have lost fat and muscle weight, putting them at risk of nutritional health problems.

Some other ways to track your nutritional health

Body mass index

Body mass index (BMI) is a commonly used assessment to determine whether your weight is helpful to your health. It was based on American health insurance statistics and, although a useful measurement, only looks at weight and height: it doesn't look at changes in body weight or assessment of body composition. The changes in body composition – muscle and fat – are probably the most important nutritional consideration in people who have either lost muscle or who have gained fat weight. Although a useful indicator of nutritional health, the BMI doesn't measure shape changes.

This can be misleading, as the absolute BMI number may present someone as being at a normal weight or even a higher than ideal weight when in fact that person may be malnourished because of the total amount of weight lost since starting treatment. For example, someone who started treatment at a weight of 110 kg (244 lb, or 17.3 stone), is 1.7 m (5 ft 6 in) tall and has lost 20 kg (44 lb, or 3 stone) in the past three months would have a BMI of 31. This as an absolute measure suggests being overweight or obese; however, the loss of nearly 20 per cent of total body weight in such a short period owing to difficulties in eating would suggest this person is at a higher risk of nutritional depletion and the associated complications of malnutrition. This is why, in addition to checking the absolute weight and a BMI during the treatment period, it is equally important to put this into context against the total weight changes of recent months.

You can assess your BMI using the chart in Figure 3.1.

Percentage weight loss

Another simple way to assess nutritional status is to look at the weight a person may have lost or gained over a certain time period as a percentage of total body weight. This will give a more accurate indication of what is happening to the body shape at the moment.

$$\text{Percentage weight loss} = \frac{\text{usual weight (kg)} - \text{current weight (kg)}}{\text{usual weight (kg)}} \times 100$$

For example, if a person's usual weight is 80 kg and six months later it is 65 kg:

$$\text{Percentage weight loss} = \frac{80 - 65}{80} \times 100 = 18.75\%$$

This would be considered a significant weight loss, with probable nutritional consequences. Although many people might like a lower weight of 65 kg (10 stone), it is important to realize that significant amounts of unintentional weight loss are associated with reduced prognosis and nutrition-related complications.

It can also be easy to miss small amounts of weight loss. For example a 5 per cent weight loss in a 50 kg (8 stone) person is a loss of just 2.5 kg (4.5 lb). Regularly checking your weight and other measurements of nutrition status helps to ensure changes are picked up and acted upon sooner rather than later.

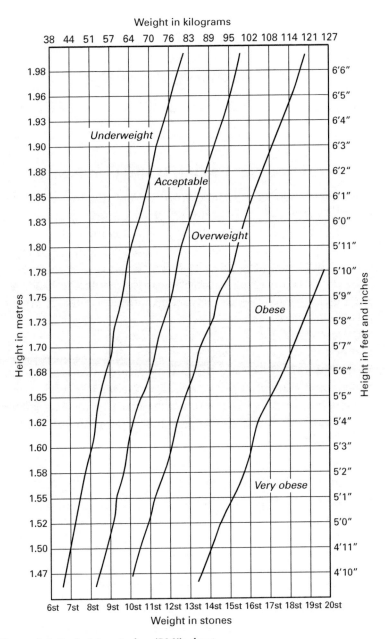

Figure 3.1 Body Mass Index (BMI) chart

Taken from Dr Robert Povey, Dr Claire Hallas and Dr Rachel Povey, *Living with a Heart Bypass*, London, Sheldon Press, 2006, p. 82.

4

Cancer treatments:
what to expect and how to prepare

How cancer treatments affect nutrition

Once cancer has been diagnosed, there are usually several decisions to be made about the most effective course of treatment. This may involve surgery, chemotherapy, radiotherapy and other types of treatment. Essential as they are to the successful treatment of cancer, they often have side effects which can contribute to eating problems. Certain types of surgery, particularly to the head, neck and digestive tract, can also impact on nutritional intake. More on this in Chapter 6.

Cancer treatments by their very nature are designed to target and destroy cancer cells, yet in doing this they also cause damage to healthy cells, especially the faster-growing cells, such as those which line the mouth, tongue and digestive tract. It is the damage to these healthy cells that can sometimes make eating and enjoying your usual food more challenging. Some of the common side effects can include:

- a sore mouth
- changes to saliva (becomes thicker)
- taste changes ranging from loss of taste to metallic flavours
- reflux
- nausea
- vomiting
- problems with your bowels
- difficulty absorbing and tolerating certain foods.

Fortunately there are many medications and other strategies your clinical team can recommend. In addition, oncology dietitians, along with other clinical team members, can support you with specialist advice, which can be a big help. Don't forget: however unpleasant your side effects may be, the likelihood is that we have come across them before, and that we know a number of ways in which they might be tackled. So, again, do ask!

Cancer treatments and possible nutritional effects

There are many types and combinations of treatment. It is very important to remember that you are an individual with a particular type of cancer (bear in mind there are over 200 types) and a specific treatment will be prescribed just for you.

The main types of treatment are:

- chemotherapy
- radiotherapy
- surgery
- hormonal therapies
- biological therapies.

Although in what follows I outline how some of the common side effects may affect your nutritional health, it is important to discuss this in detail with your healthcare support team. Not everyone responds to treatments in the same way. It makes absolutely no sense to take nutritional advice from well-intentioned friends or family members who happen to know someone else with cancer, as most likely the other person's type and experience will be completely different from yours.

Chemotherapy

Chemotherapy works by intercepting and blocking the cancer cell growth and reproduction processes. This causes them to die off. It can be given in many ways, including in tablet form or via injection. There are over 50 different types of chemotherapy, given either as individual agents or in various combinations. It may also be used in combination with surgery, radiotherapy or other treatments.

As chemotherapy travels through the bloodstream it can reach cancer cells anywhere in the body, but along the way it often also damages some of the healthy cells. Those most likely to be affected are the bone marrow (which makes blood cells), the hair, the skin, the mouth and the digestive tract. However, while the cancer cells die off, the healthy cells will over time regenerate and grow back to normal function. Your nutritional health can make an important contribution to this.

Although not everyone experiences them, chemotherapy can cause various side effects depending on which drug (or combination of drugs) is used.

The common side effects of chemotherapy

The following are all common side effects of chemotherapy that can affect your usual eating patterns:

- loss of appetite
- taste changes
- sore mouth, mouth ulcers
- saliva changes, thick viscous saliva
- nausea and vomiting
- bowel changes – diarrhoea, constipation
- fatigue
- low mood
- weight changes (loss or gain)
- low white blood cell counts or immune compromise, which increases risks of infection.

Chemotherapy's impact on the blood

Chemotherapy can cause a decrease in your red blood cells (anaemia). Anaemia can also be caused by radiation, by cancer itself or by deficiency of a nutrient such as iron, folate or vitamin B12. One way to help your red blood cell count is to eat a nutritious diet that includes lots of lean protein foods along with enough calories. If you lose weight, your body uses your muscles, red blood cells and other organs, which it converts into the energy the body needs to continue to function. If your blood count becomes too low your doctor will also look at medical ways to improve it, but you should not start supplements unless advised to do so. If you have low levels of iron please refer to Chapter 5 for further ways to boost your dietary intake.

Chemotherapy can also cause a drop in the white blood cells that fight off infections and protect the body from foodborne illnesses. This is called neutropenia. You may hear your team describe you as neutropenic, which means that your immune system is weaker than usual and you are at a higher risk of infection or food poisoning. Although there are no foods you can eat to protect against neutropenia, it is important to follow the food safety guidelines in Chapter 8 (see page 118).

What to eat and how to prepare for your chemotherapy treatment day

Do not come into treatment on an empty stomach. Try to eat a good breakfast, such as cereal with milk and fruit, or toast and an egg with a glass of fruit juice.

If you are travelling a long distance to your treatment centre, bring a snack with you, such as a smoothie drink, cereal bar or nuts and dried fruit. If you bring foods that require refrigeration you should pack them in a cooler bag.

Depending on the catering options at your treatment centre, you may also want to bring in some bigger snacks or your lunch. It is best to include some lean protein, such as a sandwich or pitta containing chicken, lean ham, tuna, cheese or egg, or you could try peanut butter. You could also bring a small thermos flask of a hearty soup if you are having difficulty chewing and swallowing whole foods. Other options are soft milk puddings, small tins of stewed fruit, or pasta salad.

Also look at my Food Fix suggestions in Chapters 6 and 7 if you are having specific symptoms such as bowel problems or nausea.

Alternatively you may be able to buy some food on your way to treatment, perhaps treating yourself to a delicious sandwich, soup, tart, milkshake, yoghurt or whatever you fancy from one of the many high street food outlets or supermarkets such as Marks & Spencer, Tesco, Waitrose, Sainsbury's, etc.

Another option that might be worth trying is one of the nutritional sip feed drinks such as Ensure Plus, Fortisip or Resource (see Chapter 7). Sometimes sipping on these drinks is easier than eating, and you may be able to try them at your treatment centre if you talk to your nurse or the dietitian.

Avoid heavy, fried or greasy food if you are not feeling well. It is also best to avoid foods with a pungent aroma. Also be mindful of people around you on treatment day. It is best to leave foods with strong smells out of the treatment suite as others near you may be feeling unwell.

Ensure you drink two litres of water on and after your treatment day. This is important to flush your system out. If you find drinking water difficult, you can flavour it with a cordial or barley water such as elderflower, lemon or orange. Alternatively you can use sports drinks such as Lucozade or Gatorade. This is helpful if you are having trouble with your appetite.

Take extra care with food hygiene. Keep away from salad or buffet bars. Ensure all food has been refrigerated properly, and avoid foods with live cultures or anything unpasteurized. Refer to the food safety guidelines on page 120.

If you are experiencing side effects I cannot stress enough the importance of discussing these with your treatment suite nurses or your doctor. It is essential that you raise any problems to help prevent more serious complications such as blood electrolyte changes, dehydration, continuing weight loss or infections. There are many effective medicines to deal with nausea, vomiting, reflux, bowel changes and mouth and skin problems. It is also important to inform the doctors or nurses who are looking after you if you have found a particular medicine to be unhelpful or if your problem has continued. You may need a change in the dose or another medicine altogether. Too often I meet people who have lost weight or had a terrible time with nausea or bowel problems. When I ask about the medication they were prescribed they often say that it didn't seem to work or that they didn't want to take too many medicines. They also do not want to bother their busy doctor or the flat-out nurses and instead go on suffering in silence. Often, side effects do not go away like a headache, and it is better to speak up sooner rather than later if you are having any difficulties. Most centres also provide an after-hours number to call. When I am told about continuing nausea or the like, I will either tell the patient to contact his or her doctor straightaway or will make the contact myself. Usually the doctor is able to recommend a more suitable alternative that can help resolve this and save a lot of unnecessary pain or distress.

Treat yourself to something special. Go for the best quality food options you can – maybe you can tempt yourself with a lovely piece of cheddar from a cheese shop or deli counter rather than the usual sliced or block options, and a special crispbread to go with it. You may also like a delicious piece of cake or scone, or a cupcake that will melt in your mouth.

If you have been following a special diet to help lower your cholesterol or manage diabetes, it is important to know whether restricting your diet is important during the time you are in treatment, especially if you are having trouble eating. Do discuss this with your doctor or dietitian.

Radiotherapy

Radiotherapy, or radiation therapy uses directed rays of radiation to destroy the DNA of cancer cells, which prevents them from growing and multiplying. Although it is targeted at the cancer cells it may also hit healthy cells, and this can contribute to side effects. The therapy is delivered in small consecutive doses, usually for two to ten weeks, and is commonly used to treat cancers of the breast, head, neck, brain and colon. It is also often used in combination with other types of treatment such as chemotherapy (chemoradiation) and surgery. Not all cancers respond to radiotherapy.

Nutritional side effects of radiotherapy

The nutritional side effects of radiotherapy depend on the area being treated, the dose and the duration of treatment. They also depend on whether the therapy is used in combination with other treatments such as chemotherapy. Typically, side effects present at around two to three weeks into treatment and can last around two to six weeks after treatment has finished. The main side effects which can impact on nutritional health are those which affect the mouth region, including mouth ulcers and saliva and taste changes. The other region prone to side effects is in the gastrointestinal tract. Table 4.1 lists some common nutritional side effects of radiotherapy.

How can I prepare for my radiotherapy?

Do refer to the suggestions for preparing for chemotherapy on page 37. However, as the appointments for radiotherapy are usually frequent and sequential, you may need to take time to stock up and be organized, so that you are ready to bring some food supplies each day. If you are experiencing difficulties, you may need to talk

Table 4.1 Common nutritional side effects of radiotherapy

Area of treatment	Possible side effects affecting nutrition
Brain, spinal cord	Nausea, vomiting, fatigue, loss or increased appetite
Head and neck (tongue, larynx (voice box), tonsils, salivary glands, nose area)	Sore mouth and throat, difficulties or pain with swallowing, taste and smell changes, thick or sticky saliva, loss of appetite, fatigue
Lung, oesophagus, breast	Sore throat, difficulties swallowing, heartburn or reflux, fatigue and loss of appetite
Stomach, large or small bowel, pelvic region, cervix, uterus or ovaries, rectum, pancreas, prostate	Nausea, vomiting, diarrhoea, gas, bloating, lactose intolerance, loss of appetite, changes in bladder function, fatigue

to your doctor or nurse or the dietitian about taking some extra sip feed nutrition drinks, or other options, to ensure you are able to receive enough nutrition during your treatment.

Surgery

Surgery is often the most important component of treatments for many cancers. It can be used to remove cancerous tissues or to help reduce tumour size. Depending on the type and stage of the cancer, treatment may also include chemotherapy and radiotherapy either before the surgery (neo-adjuvant) or after it (adjuvant).

Nutrition-related side effects of surgery

As with all surgery, the body experiences a degree of stress and needs to go through a healing and recovery process. Some surgical procedures can affect nutrient absorption or the ability to eat normally. Surgery to the head and neck region is often associated with difficulties with chewing and swallowing due to pain, swelling or the removal of parts of the mouth and throat during the surgery. Specific nutritional guidance is often prescribed, and at times this may require extra support with a feeding tube.

Surgery to the gastrointestinal tract may also affect the ability to absorb nutrients. Surgery on the stomach, the pancreas and the small and large bowel has the potential to impact on the normal absorption of food nutrients including fat, carbohydrate, protein, vitamins and minerals. Fluid, electrolyte balance and fibre digestion also need to be considered in surgery to the large bowel area.

How can I prepare for surgery?

Aim for a high protein, high energy diet to build up your strength. If you are having difficulty eating or swallowing, consider taking high protein milkshakes or, if you can manage them, soft or puréed foods.

After surgery it is important to know whether your ability to eat or digest may be affected. Again, this is something to discuss with your doctor or cancer dietitian.

Practical preparation:

- Fill the refrigerator, cupboard and freezer with nourishing foods. Make sure to include items you can eat even when you feel sick (see Chapter 6 for suggestions on combating nausea).
- Stock up on foods that need little or no cooking, such as frozen dinners and ready-to-eat cooked foods. Frozen soups are an excellent idea.
- Cook some foods ahead of time and freeze in meal-sized portions.
- Ask friends or family to help you shop and cook during treatment. Maybe a friend can set up a schedule of tasks that need to be done and people who are willing to do them.
- Talk with your doctor, nurse or dietitian about what to expect. See the lists of foods and drinks that can help with many types of eating problems (Chapter 6).

Hormonal therapies

Hormonal therapies work to block or dilute certain hormones that help drive the growth of particular hormone-responsive cancer cells. The main use for hormonal therapies is in certain hormone-positive types of breast and prostate cancer. There are many different types of hormonal therapies and these can have some side effects which impact on nutritional health. Possible side effects can include fatigue, early onset menopause and increased risk of osteoporosis, and some individuals find they are prone to some weight gain and mood changes. A healthier approach to your diet is recommended, together with some regular exercise, as well as making any adjustments you need to mitigate any specific side effects that may occur. At times these may include nausea or a sore mouth, and some treatments may affect bowel function. These symptoms are usually temporary and resolve after treatment.

Biological therapies

Biological therapies are an emerging group of cancer treatments, many of which are in the trial phase. They are treatments which utilize various defence type substances or chemicals that occur naturally and work as part of the immune or cell regulation systems. They work to either attack or control the growth of cancer cells, or can be used to help individuals tolerate more potent doses of other cancer treatments. The way they work at the cell level is very specific to the type of biological therapy, although broadly they work at a specific site on the cancer cell, helping to block the blood supply to these cells or impeding the way these cells interact and communicate to facilitate their ongoing growth.

There are many types of biological treatments and the side effects vary depending on the type of biological treatment you are to receive.

Again, it will be best to discuss with your doctor or nurse specialist how the treatment you have been recommended will work in your body, and at this time the side effects will also be discussed at the individual level. However, some of the broad-brush possibilities which may concern your nutritional health include fatigue, nausea, a sore mouth, bowel habit changes, loss of appetite and some impacts on your blood counts.

5

Preparing for treatment at home: ways to eat well (with recipes)

Working out your daily energy and nutrient allowances

When you have cancer, you may need more protein and more calories.

When working out what amounts of energy and nutrients you need during your day, it can be helpful to think of food nutrients as a currency. While the normal currency used is calories or kilojoules, consider each of the key food nutrients as being worth a certain amount of money. If you are losing weight and having a difficult time, you need to try to eat more to increase the savings you have in the bank. These savings will be then available for you to spend on each of the body's key functions, including:

- brain function
- immune system function
- mobility
- extra healing
- cellular repair
- energy to go out.

If you find you are putting on extra, unwanted pounds, keep to a stricter budget that focuses on just including the foods that provide the most nutrient value, such as fruits, vegetables, lean proteins and wholegrains, without too many high-fat, sugar or alcohol purchases. Now you can plan the shopping either to build up the bank or to try and keep a tighter control on the total daily spend to balance the energy books.

Energy intake = energy for essential body function + energy for stress and repair + energy for activity or exercise

The macronutrient allowances

The main food nutrients which provide energy for body function, repair and activity are called macronutrients. Ensuring you are taking enough of these should be the first step in any dietary plan.

The energy allowances of the macronutrients are as follows:

- carbohydrates: 4 kcal/g
- protein: 4 kcal/g
- fat: 9 kcal/g
- alcohol: 7 kcal/g
- fibre: a small amount of energy.

Carbohydrates

Carbohydrates form the body's major provider of energy. This is a group that I would like to champion as many people, when considering their dietary needs, forget that carbohydrates give the body the fuel it needs for physical activity and proper organ function. They are a valuable source of many nutrients for health, including vitamins, minerals, wholegrains and fibre.

The best sources of carbohydrates include fruits, vegetables and wholegrains – these also supply the body's cells with many of the essential vitamins and minerals, fibre and phytonutrients ('fight-o-nutrients': important chemicals found in plants; more about them later in this chapter and in Chapter 10).

Wholegrains or foods made from them contain all the essential parts and naturally occurring nutrients of the entire grain seed. Wholegrains are found in cereals, breads, flours and crackers. Some wholegrains, such as quinoa, brown rice or barley, can be used as side dishes or part of an entrée. When choosing a wholegrain product, look for terms such as 'wholegrain', 'stone ground', 'whole ground', 'wholewheat flour', 'whole-oat flour' or 'whole-rye flour'.

What about slow- or fast-release carbohydrates?

The Glycaemic Index (GI) or Glycaemic Load (GL) concept can be used to select carbohydrates to improve satiety and blood sugar control. The types of carbohydrates which are best in helping with unwanted weight gain, blood sugar control, hunger pangs or low energy are the lower GI or slower-release type carbohydrates.

Table 5.1 Fast- and slow-release carbohydrates

Fast-release carbohydrates or higher GI (lower satiety)	Slow-release carbohydrates or lower GI (higher satiety)
Well-cooked or fresh pasta	Durum wheat pasta cooked *al dente*
Cornflakes, Rice Krispies, Frosties, Coco Pops, etc.	All-Bran, natural muesli made with whole oats, whole oat porridge
Large well-cooked or mashed potato	Baby or new potatoes cooked whole in the jacket
Quick-cook oats	Whole oats or pinhead type oats, oat groats
White or wholemeal bread	Wholegrain or soya and linseed bread
Soft drinks, cordials, fruit juice	Milk, yoghurt
Jasmine or short-grain rice	Basmati or brown rice
Rice or corn cakes	Ryvita crispbreads

Basically, as these foods are mostly wholegrain or unprocessed grain or cereal type foods, the body takes longer to break them down. In addition to helping you feel full for longer, the energy they provide tends to last for around two to three hours.

The higher GI or fast-release carbohydrates are the ones which are either cooked more or processed more, or are in more broken-down form. These give a quicker hit of energy and tend not to fill you up as much. They may be better if you are experiencing early satiety or are losing weight. Table 5.1 lists some slow- and fast-release carbohydrates.

The relevance of the slow or fast carbohydrate choices in treatment

While the GI (slow or fast) is a well-researched concept, there are a number of confounding factors and the choices can be hard to apply to real meals.

The best advice I can give is to use the GI concept either to eat more of the foods that fill you up, or to eat more of the foods that are easy to eat and don't cause as much of a problem with early satiety. It is best only to apply the GI concept to grain- or cereal-based carbohydrate foods including pasta, bread, potatoes, beverages and breakfast cereal choices. It is important not to worry about the GI with fruit and vegetables as, owing to the lower carbohydrate content of these foods, the difference is negligible and it is always better to try to get in as many different fruit and vegetable colours as you can.

Examples of how to modify recipes for either a slow or faster release of carbohydrate energy

It is very easy to adjust your old recipes from high GI to low GI. To slow down the rate of carbohydrate release in any type of baked goods you can adjust and switch the ingredients to incorporate more of the following: apple, fructose sugar, oats, All-Bran, linseeds, etc.

For savoury casserole-type meals, try adding a small tin of lentils to your mince; use sweet potatoes instead of normal potatoes in a stew, curry or roast dinner and even for mashed potato. There are many recipe books available now that have low GI recipes.

Low GI or high satiety bran muffins (also very high fibre)

This recipe is a good example of eating for sustained slow-release energy, giving you an excellent blood sugar control and energy for three hours after eating.

NOTE: This batter has to stand overnight.

2 eggs
60 ml (4 tablesp) rapeseed oil
375 ml (1½ cups) flour, sifted before measuring
1 large grated apple
5 ml (1 teasp) ground cinnamon
5 ml (1 teasp) vanilla essence
150 g (1 cup) soft brown sugar (could use fructose sugar)

250 ml (1 cup) oat bran, pressed down into the cup
500 ml (2 cups) digestive bran
15 ml (1 tablesp) bicarbonate of soda
2 ml (½ teasp) salt
250 ml (1 cup) sultanas
500 ml (2 cups) low-fat milk

Beat together the eggs, sugar and oil. Add all the dry ingredients, the grated apple and the sultanas. Mix thoroughly, lifting the mixture a few times with the spoon to incorporate air. Mix the milk and vanilla and add to the flour mixture. Stir until well blended, but do not over-mix. Leave overnight in the refrigerator. When ready to bake, stir and drop into muffin pans and bake at 180° C/170° C fan/350° F/Gas Mark 4 for 15 minutes. Makes 24 large muffins.

This mixture can be kept in the refrigerator for up to 30 days. Do not freeze the batter, but baked muffins freeze very well.

High GI or lower satiety blueberry and banana muffins

Using more of the refined types of flours and sugar with ripe or more tropical fruits generally means the GI is higher and the food processed by the body at a quicker rate.

2½ cups self-raising flour	¾ cup brown sugar
1 tablespoon caster sugar	1 teaspoon vanilla extract
¾ cup milk	½ cup frozen blueberries
1 egg, lightly beaten	2 ripe bananas, mashed
½ cup vegetable oil	

Preheat oven to 190°C/170°C fan/375°F/Gas Mark 5. Line a 12-hole muffin pan with paper cases. Combine the flour, caster sugar and brown sugar in a bowl. Make a well in the centre and add the milk, egg, oil and vanilla. Mix until just combined. Fold in the blueberries and bananas. Spoon mixture evenly between paper cases. Bake for 20 to 22 minutes or until golden and just firm to touch. Stand in pan for 5 minutes. Transfer to a wire rack to cool.

Muffins are best served on the day of cooking. Avoid over-mixing the muffin batter or it results in a tough texture.

Protein

Protein needs to be a focus nutrient for people with cancer. Cancer does take it out of you, along with the treatments, and surgery can place quite a bit of stress on the body. Enough protein, and a better quality of protein, can increase the rate of tissue repair and boost the immune system, making recovery time quicker and easier.

In addition to eating regular bite-sized portions of protein-rich foods throughout the day, include more of the higher quality protein sources, which provide more of the specific tissue building blocks or amino acids that the body uses for growth and repair.

It is also important to know that if your energy budgets are not being met or if you are losing weight, the protein you eat will need to be put into the fuel tank and used as a basic energy source. This means the rate of growth and repair is generally sluggish.

During treatment, eat more high biological value proteins, where the amino acid profile is a closer match to what the body needs more of at this time.

- High biological value proteins include fish, poultry, lean red meat, eggs, dairy products and whey-based protein (supplements).
- Other good protein sources, although not as high in their biological value scores, are nuts and nut butters, dried beans, peas and lentils, and soy foods. These are good supplement protein foods.

A note on red meat

Lean red meat is a very high quality type of protein. It contains a potent source of iron and is often a food the body needs more of during treatment. This is an example of a food that should generally not be restricted during the treatment phase, although I do encourage choices which are lean, come from a good source and are from a better quality cut. The guidelines on red meat are intended for those trying to prevent their first cancer or who have finished treatment and are eating well to prevent a future recurrence. They are not intended for individuals, particularly those who might be struggling with their diet, during the active treatment stage.

A note on dairy products

Many people give up dairy foods when they find out they have cancer, especially women with breast cancer. I certainly do not recommend this and would advise anyone who has taken this step to revisit the evidence behind this hot issue. (For more information, see Chapter 9, page 124.)

How much protein needs to be eaten?

Generally, individuals who are well and not experiencing any additional problems should aim for around 0.8–1.0 g of protein per kilogram of body weight. This would be around 60–75 g/day of protein for a 75 kg (12 stone) person.

However, if you are in treatment, more active and trying to build muscle, then you may need to increase your protein intake towards 1.2–2 g per kilogram of body weight. At the upper end this would be around 135–150 g of protein for the same 75 kg (12 stone) person.

These broad-brush guidelines have been taken from published data on protein needs for healthy individuals, athletes and people who are experiencing illness or stress. They are only suitable if you have no problems with your liver or kidney function.

A person who is cachexic and losing weight has a very challenging protein requirement of 1.8–2.0 g per kilogram of body weight, a target that can be more difficult to reach as often appetite is poor. This is when it might be easier to use supplements such as protein powders. The cheapest protein powder is skimmed milk powder and it is easy to add to most meals.

Table 5.2 lists foods providing approximately 10 g of protein from both higher and lower quality types of protein.

Table 5.2 Foods providing approximately 10 g of protein from both higher and lower quality types of protein

Animal (high-value protein)	Plant
2 small eggs	4 slices wholemeal bread
30 g (1½) slices low-fat cheese	3 cups wholegrain cereal
250 ml (1 cup) low-fat milk	2 cups cooked pasta
70 g cottage cheese	3 cups cooked rice
30 g lean chicken or beef or pork	¾ cup lentils or kidney beans
50 g grilled fish	200 g baked beans
50 g tuna or salmon	½ cup tofu
200 g low-fat yoghurt	60 g nuts or seeds
¼ cup parmesan cheese, grated	300 ml soy milk
2 cups ice cream	100 g soy meat or Quorn
180 g Greek yoghurt	2 tablespoons peanut butter
¼ cup skimmed milk powder	⅓ cup edamame (soy beans)
30 g canned tuna	

1–2 scoops protein powder (There are many options for protein powders and you can discuss with your doctor or dietitian the most suitable one and the sorts of amounts you should be aiming for. The amount of protein per serving is detailed in the nutrition panel on the packet.)

Protein distribution

Rather than a big slab of chicken, fish or meat at the end of the day, it is better to spread protein intake in more bite-size chunks over the day.

High protein breakfast

Protein pancakes

This is a good recipe for the day of treatment.

1 egg	*Blueberries*
5 egg whites	*Oil spray for frying (or use a non-*
120 g oats	*stick pan)*
Honey or maple syrup	

Whisk together egg whites and oats. Pour mixture into hot pan. Turn when it starts to bubble. Serve with honey or maple syrup and blueberries.

What a yummy way to boost the morning, with 38 g of protein, of which 25 g is high-value protein.

Fats

Despite its bad press, fat has an important role in treatment nutrition, especially if you are trying to boost or maintain your weight and muscle levels. Omega 3 fatty acids can also help reduce inflammation and boost memory and mood.

Fats and oils are made of fatty acids and serve as a rich source of energy for the body. The body breaks down fats and uses them to store energy and to insulate body tissues, transporting some types of fat-soluble vitamins through the blood. Low mood is also associated with very low-fat diets and inadequate intakes of omega 3 fatty acids, an important fat for the body, which is found in oily fish, rapeseed, linseeds and, to a lesser degree, olive oil.

You may have heard that some fats are better for you than others. While heart health shouldn't be the main focus when you are in treatment for cancer, it is good to keep it on the radar, especially if you are otherwise well. I would suggest using a delicious olive oil on salads or bread, and cooking with rapeseed oils, nut oils, hemp oils and other vegetable-based margarines or oils. It can be a good idea to mix your oils around, although when you are not well it is hard to beat the taste of real butter. I generally tell people to worry about cholesterol and the like once they have finished treatment, unless it is a major health priority to them. Quite often I find myself gently persuading gorgeous – but little – older ladies that really the cholesterol concern is not that important to them at this time. It certainly has been a public health message that many people get stuck on, but it is not normally one of the main nutritional priorities during the treatment phase unless you are otherwise advised by your doctor or you have a cancer like prostate and some colon cancers, which are often related to heart health and excessive amounts of weight.

Different types of fat

- Mono-unsaturated fats are found mainly in vegetable oils like olive, rapeseed and peanut oils.
- Polyunsaturated fats are found mainly in vegetable oils like safflower, sunflower, corn and flaxseed. They are also the main fats found in seafood.
- Saturated fats are mainly in animal sources like meat and poultry, cream or whole-fat milk, cheese and butter. Some vegetable oils, like coconut, palm kernel and palm oil, are saturated. After treatment it is important to know that saturated fats can raise cholesterol and increase your risk of heart disease. Less than 10 per cent of your calories should come from saturated fat. People on hormonal treatment can have a higher risk of heart disease further down the track.
- Trans-fatty acids are formed when vegetable oils are processed into margarine or shortening. Sources of trans-fats include snack foods and baked goods made with partially hydrogenated vegetable oil or vegetable shortening. They can raise bad cholesterol and lower good cholesterol; try to eliminate them from your diet, although this is not necessarily the biggest priority during the treatment phase.

A note on fish oils

High doses of the fish oil EPA (2 g/day) can act as an anti-inflammatory, and there is a moderate amount of evidence to suggest that a daily dose may reduce the loss of appetite often experienced with more advanced cancers. It should be noted that fish oils should not be taken if you are receiving any platin-based chemotherapy agents. If you are unsure, check with your doctor or nurse specialist.

Fibre

Fibre is the part of plant foods that the body cannot digest. There are two types:

- Insoluble fibre provides the bulk, and this is important to move food waste out of the body quickly, acting like a big broom. Insoluble fibre sources include wholegrain cereal foods such as bread, wholegrain crispbreads, higher-fibre breakfast cereals (look at the fibre levels on the side of the packet), brown rice, wholemeal pasta, popcorn, fruit skins and pips.
- Soluble fibre binds with water in the stool to help keep stools soft, and this type of fibre is more fermentable. Soluble fibre sources include fruit, legumes, vegetables and oats.

For bowel function a good balance between both types of fibre throughout the day is important.

If you are experiencing difficulties with sluggish bowels, it may be worth discussing with your doctor or clinic whether the gradual build-up of your insoluble and soluble fibre intakes is safe and appropriate for you. Also see the Food Fix ideas in Chapter 7 on diet tips for constipation. However, please note that in some situations constipation is not related to diet and a high-fibre diet can further aggravate the situation. This needs to be discussed with your doctor.

If you are experiencing wind and bloating, start by checking you are not overdoing the fruit and vegetable intake. Quite often this is an issue for individuals who move from ground zero to eating fruits and vegetables until they are coming out of their ears!

Although we encourage lots of variety and colours in your diet, during treatment it can be harder for the body to manage large volumes of these foods, especially when this has not been the normal dietary practice. In such situations, it's best to start with four to five servings of fruit and vegetables a day and slowly build up.

Other foods which can affect bloating are referred to as the more fermentable types or higher FODMAP foods. FODMAP is an acronym standing for a group of carbohydrates which are poorly digested plant residues particularly fermentable in the large bowel. The diet can be used to assess whether reducing these types of foods can help in the management of what are referred to as functional gastrointestinal symptoms, which may include bloating, excessive wind, pain and continuing changes in bowel habit such as diarrhoea or constipation. The diet should be worked out in consultation with a gastroenterologist and a specialist dietitian; however, you can experiment with cutting out foods such as onions, garlic, high fructose fruits such as apples and pears, pulses, sorbitol or xylitol-containing mints or gums.

Water

It is always important to consume enough water so that you strike the balance between dehydration and over-hydration. Too much water can cause hyponatremia, a life-threatening drop in your sodium levels. Smaller, less active women are at a higher risk of taking in too much water.

We all know that water and liquids or fluids are vital to health and that our cells need water to function. During treatment, taking in enough fluid is also important to help flush out the drugs from the system once they have finished working. Being slightly dehydrated – by as little as 1 to 2 per cent – can affect how you feel and function. Studies indicate that if you are dehydrated by 2 per cent or more, you will not perform as well as if you were hydrated. This is key if you are losing fluids through vomiting or diarrhoea.

How much water to drink

In general, around six to eight glasses of fluid are recommended a day. This should include water, although other fluids such as tea, coffee, juices and cordials all contribute. If you are having chemotherapy, you are advised to try to take in two litres a day, although this can be difficult and may contribute to waking during the night, which is not helpful if fatigue is a problem. It is certainly better to try to take more of this fluid earlier in the day. One way to gauge whether you are drinking enough is to observe the colour of your urine. Some drugs and vitamins may affect the colour, but you should be aiming for pale yellow to straw. Dark-coloured urine can be an indication of dehydration. Some sport nutritionists have put together a clever iPhone app called Ipee Daily. This app provides a Dulux-type colour chart to track the colour of your urine!

Finally, if you are unable to keep fluids down or are experiencing extreme diarrhoea, contact your clinic immediately.

Vitamins and minerals

Although vitamins and minerals are essential for good health, the body only needs small amounts. Quite often there is a disproportionate focus on the need for enough or extra vitamins and minerals, which probably has something to do with aggressive supplement company promotions.

Vitamins and minerals are found naturally in food, and in general a person who eats a balanced and varied diet with enough calories and protein gets plenty. There are, of course, times when this is difficult in the treatment phase, and in such instances it would be appropriate to discuss the use of a low-dose multi-vitamin and mineral supplement with your medical advisers.

What I do want to caution you against is the practice of megadosing. Often, people with cancer are advised to take – or believe they need – large amounts of vitamins, minerals and other dietary supplements to try to boost everything from their energy levels to their immune system. They may even believe that these supplements can destroy cancer cells. This is not the case; in fact, taking larger doses of supplements can be harmful and there are many studies which associate this practice with a higher incidence of cancer. Large doses of some vitamins and minerals are also known to be likely to impact on the effectiveness of chemotherapy and radiation therapy.

The most prudent advice is to aim to eat enough of a variety of foods to provide for your requirements. If you are concerned, and if your oncologist agrees, talk to your pharmacist about selecting a supplement with no more than 100 per cent of the daily value (DV) of vitamins and minerals and one with a lower level of iron (unless your doctor has found your iron to be low and would generally advise an appropriate level of iron supplementation).

Phytonutrients or phytochemicals

These are plant compounds like carotenoids, lycopene, resveratrol and phytosterols that are thought to have health-protecting qualities. They are found in plant products such as fruits, vegetables and teas. Pill or supplement forms of phytochemicals have not been shown to be as helpful as eating the foods that contain them. I have included more detail on this in Chapter 10 (see page 135).

Antioxidants

Among the focus phytonutrients in the cancer arena are antioxidants, as there is widespread interest in their potential to attack and block free radicals, considered to be harmful molecules that cause damage to normal healthy cells.

The main antioxidants of interest have included vitamins A, C and E, selenium and zinc, and some enzymes. However, as with many areas in nutrition, once something is found to be positive people somehow become convinced that bucket-loads must be much better than ordinary moderate amounts. This enthusiasm is fuelled by companies who package them as supplements, and they start to appear in weird and wonderful forms, to be loaded into the body throughout the day, whether in the form of a pill or powder or by having that juicer going 24/7. The number of times I have inwardly cringed when I hear of people trying to down litres of broccoli juice and other horrible-looking green powder mixes that claim the wonders of being 'super-green'! I remember meeting one lady who was drinking around two litres of broccoli, cabbage and beetroot juice a day. I could not imagine having to clean a juicer every day after that mix.

It is understandable that people want to do all they can to fight cancer. However, what needs to be recognized is that we just do not fully understand the complex nature of cellular function. While we have labelled the free radical action as a bad thing, it may in fact be a good thing for our cells. Perhaps the free radicals help cull cells which are not functioning as well as they should, and perhaps our amazing body does have a better idea of cell regulation than many of the quasi-nutritionists who advocate the need for copious amounts of super-greens and the like, without any strong evidence to show that the effort involved in downing all these extras is in fact helping. Or, even more importantly, that they are not doing more harm than good.

If you want to take in more antioxidants, what we strongly recommend is that you try to eat a variety of fruits and vegetables, which are also good sources of other valuable nutrients, as well as fibre. In most clinics I know, people are not advised to take extra and certainly not large doses of antioxidant supplements or vitamin-enhanced foods or liquids. This is because of their potential to interact and compete with the tasks assigned to the chemo- or radiotherapy. Talk with your doctor or dietitian about finding a safe way to enjoy an adequate intake of antioxidants in your diet. (See also Chapter 10.) There is nothing wrong with having some food boosters to help you out during the treatment stage, just as long as the food priorities are in the right order.

Putting it all together

Figure 5.1, the Eatwell Plate, shows recommendations for healthy, balanced eating. It can be a good starting point if you are well and not experiencing too many difficulties with your diet. However, your plate may need to look quite different, with more emphasis on protein and dairy foods if you are struggling with your appetite and normal food intake, as in Figures 5.2 and 5.3 (see pages 57–8).

Jane's action-packed treatment foods

Milk and skimmed milk powder

Milk is an important food as it provides high amounts of protein, energy and calcium. The type of milk you choose depends on whether you are trying to 'build up' or 'hold on' to where you are. The choice is full fat or low fat, the difference being that:

- whole or full-fat milk contains about 3.5 per cent fat;
- semi-skimmed contains about 1.7 per cent fat;
- skimmed milk contains 0.1 to 0.3 per cent fat.

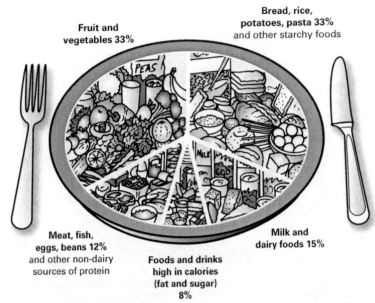

Fruit and
vegetables 33%

Bread, rice,
potatoes, pasta 33%
and other starchy foods

Meat, fish,
eggs, beans 12%
and other non-dairy
sources of protein

Foods and drinks
high in calories
(fat and sugar)
8%

Milk and
dairy foods 15%

Figure 5.1 The Eatwell Plate
Adapted from the diagram at <www.dh.gov.uk/health/2012/06/about-the-eatwell-plate/>

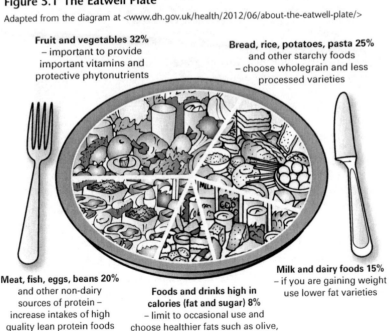

Fruit and vegetables 32%
– important to provide
important vitamins and
protective phytonutrients

Bread, rice, potatoes, pasta 25%
and other starchy foods
– choose wholegrain and less
processed varieties

Meat, fish, eggs, beans 20%
and other non-dairy
sources of protein –
increase intakes of high
quality lean protein foods

Foods and drinks high in
calories (fat and sugar) 8%
– limit to occasional use and
choose healthier fats such as olive,
rapeseed and vegetable oils

Milk and dairy foods 15%
– if you are gaining weight
use lower fat varieties

Figure 5.2 The 'high-protein' Eatwell Plate
Adapted by the author from the 'Eatwell Plate'.

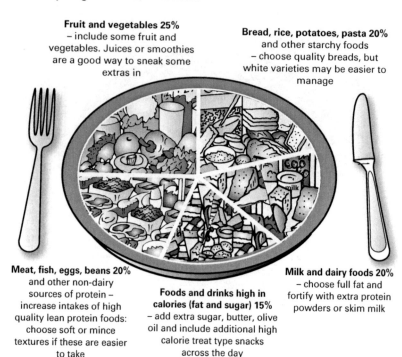

Fruit and vegetables 25%
– include some fruit and vegetables. Juices or smoothies are a good way to sneak some extras in

Bread, rice, potatoes, pasta 20%
and other starchy foods – choose quality breads, but white varieties may be easier to manage

Meat, fish, eggs, beans 20%
and other non-dairy sources of protein – increase intakes of high quality lean protein foods: choose soft or mince textures if these are easier to take

Foods and drinks high in calories (fat and sugar) 15%
– add extra sugar, butter, olive oil and include additional high calorie treat type snacks across the day

Milk and dairy foods 20%
– choose full fat and fortify with extra protein powders or skim milk

Figure 5.3 The 'build-up' Eatwell Plate
Adapted by the author from the 'Eatwell Plate'.

A lower fat content doesn't mean a lower calcium content – but low-fat milk contains less energy and lower amounts of fat-soluble vitamins unless they are fortified.

A lactose-free milk (available in the fresh dairy section of most supermarkets) or soya or other alternatives can also be used if these suit your bowel or are your personal preference. Milk can be used for cereals, home-made milkshakes, tea and coffee. It is also useful to make milk jellies, custard or other milk puddings, easy to eat if you are wanting something bland without overt food smells.

One of the easiest and most inexpensive ways to boost the protein content of your foods is to add 2–4 tablespoons of dried skimmed milk powder to a pint (450 ml) of milk. A heaped tablespoon of skimmed milk powder provides around 3 g of protein.

High protein fruity shakes

200 ml semi-skimmed milk
10 ml (2 tablesp) dried skimmed
  milk powder

Scoop of ice cream
10 ml (2 tablesp) frozen or fresh
  red berries

Put all ingredients into a jug. Blend with a hand-held blender (worth having one of these in the house). Pour into a glass and sip with a straw.

High protein muesli biscuits

Delicious as a snack or as a breakfast quick fix.

1 cup plain generic muesli
1 cup coconut
1 cup rolled oats
10 ml (2 tablesp) linseeds (best
  to add only if the bowels are
  sluggish)

½ cup raw or white sugar
¼ cup dried skimmed milk powder
180 g butter or margarine
1 tablesp honey
1 egg, lightly beaten

Combine muesli, coconut, oats, sifted flour, sugar, linseeds and powdered milk in a bowl. Melt butter and honey together. Add to mixture, then stir in egg. Drop teaspoonfuls of mixture on to lightly greased tray. Bake at 180° C/170° C fan/350° F/Gas Mark 4 for 10–15 minutes or until light golden. Cool on trays.

Eggs

Eggs are one of the most nutritious and versatile foods that a person in treatment can use. A very compact source of nutrition, they provide a potent type of protein, every vitamin except C, and a host of essential minerals including iron. Their neutral flavour can be enjoyed in a simple way or they can be dressed up with sauces and seasonings or added for an extra boost in a range of sweet and savoury dishes. They are easy to digest and the texture is soft and easy to swallow. A quick omelette or frittata or even just a poached or boiled egg is something easy and always on hand to cook. If your appetite is poor or you are struggling, try adding extra chopped egg into rice dishes (like fried rice) or mixing it into a pasta with some cheese or ham. A dish like a quiche often suits if cold food is preferred, and foods like egg custard, cake or muffins are nutritious extras when a boost is needed. Try the omega 3 boosted eggs or even quail eggs as an in-between nibble. Eggs are an ideal start to the day; a healthy filling option could be some poached eggs with grilled tomato, mushrooms and perhaps some wilted spinach, with a tasty grain or sourdough bread.

Scrambled eggs

2 eggs

5 ml (1 tablesp) single cream or milk (whatever milk you prefer)

Salt and freshly ground pepper

15 g butter or margarine

In a bowl, whisk together the eggs, milk or cream and seasoning with a fork. Melt the butter gently in a heavy-based saucepan on a low heat, until it starts to bubble slightly. Tip in the egg mixture and, using a wooden spoon, slowly and smoothly move the egg around the base of the pan until it is thick and creamy. It should look just cooked. Remove from heat and serve immediately with a piece of bread or toast.

Lemon curd

Can be used as a lovely high protein spread or dessert. The slightly tart but smooth taste often suits mouths whose taste buds are in need of a bit of a kick.

2 large lemons (adjust quantity depending on what your taste buds are doing)

85 g butter or margarine

225 g granulated sugar

3 eggs, lightly beaten

Grate lemons on the finest grater gauge, taking care not to add any of the pith. Set zest aside. Squeeze the juice from the lemons. Put lemon juice, butter, sugar and eggs into a heavy-based saucepan or double boiler and heat gently, stirring all the time, until the mixture is thick and a few large bubbles rise to the surface of the mixture. Sieve to remove any egg bits and then stir in the lemon zest. Spoon into a warmed jam jar. Will keep in the refrigerator for a week.

Lemon curd can be spread on toast, scones and pancakes, or you can add it to muffins or cakes. It goes well on ice cream, or mixed with a little custard or cream or rice puddings. It is also a great topping for cheesecake (you can buy plain cheesecake and spread it over the top).

Butter or margarine?

I would suggest that during treatment you use either butter or margarine, depending on your preference or other health needs. After treatment, you might want to switch back to margarines. I prefer those based on olive oil. Other alternatives could be spreading some avocado or hummus, or dipping your bread in a delicious olive oil with a dash of balsamic, just like the Italians. If you really prefer the taste of butter during treatment, then I would stick with a good quality butter. Extra butter can be a help if you are losing weight, but if you are gaining it is better to use it quite sparingly.

Oils

It is best to keep a few different oils in the cupboard for cooking and salad dressings and to add some extra omega 3 health benefits. I recommend rapeseed oil for cooking as its flavour is lighter and its omega 3:6 ratio is more favourable than either olive or vegetable oils. A good quality extra-virgin olive oil is best for dressing salads, although extra-virgin olive oil is not intended for frying or cooking. Other healthy oils to experiment with are walnut, macadamia, hemp and flaxseed oils. These have a slightly nutty flavour and are a good source of omega 3 fatty acids. Sesame oil is also good for added flavour in stir-fries.

Flaxseeds

Flaxseeds or linseeds are small, shiny, dark brown seeds about the size of a sesame seed. They are the richest plant source of omega 3 fatty acids, as they provided a fatty acid called alpha-linolenic acid (ALA), a building block of omega 3 oils found in fish. Flaxseeds are also rich in ligans, a type of plant oestrogen that lowers female oestrogen levels, helps the unpleasant side effects of the menopause such as flushing and has anti-tumour properties. Flaxseeds are also helpful in the management of constipation. They are very important for vegetarians or people who do not eat fish or eggs. One or two tablespoons a day is all it takes. Flaxseeds should not be taken if you have had recent bowel surgery or are having problems with diarrhoea.

Flaxseed mighty mix

½ cup linseeds or flaxseeds
1 cup oat or rice bran
½ cup linseed meal or flaxseed
  meal

½ cup almond meal or almond
  flakes
½ cup sesame seeds, toasted
½ cup psyllium husks

Mix all ingredients together. Use 1–2 tablespoons on either cereal, fruit or yoghurt daily. While this mix provides a mighty boost of fibre, protein and ALA, it may not be suitable if you need to eat less fibre or to rest your bowel.

Oily fish, including salmon, fresh tuna, mackerel and sardines

Low in saturated fat, rich in zinc and a great source of anti-inflammatory omega 3 fatty acids – there are just so many reasons to include three or four oily fish meals across the week. Fish is also an important source of protein, potassium and prostate-protecting zinc. Fish is a very versatile food as it can be eaten canned, smoked or cooked in many ways. Easy fish meals can include fish cakes or fish pie, and there can be nothing better than a quality piece of salmon pan-fried or barbecued (always put the skin of the fish on the hot grill for protection). Tinned or smoked salmon or other fish mixed with a quality tomato sauce or some Philadelphia cheese with some capers is a very easy meal.

Fish cakes

450 g fresh salmon fillets
350 g mashed potato (not too wet)
2 eggs, beaten
1 tablespoon fresh parsley
  (chopped)

Small can corn (optional)
Dried white breadcrumbs
1 red pepper, chopped
Seasoned flour
Oil for frying

Poach the salmon in a little water and let it cool. Remove the skin and break the fish into flakes. Mix salmon and potato together. Season well with salt and pepper. Add the butter, parsley and corn (if used). Add a small amount of egg if needed to bind the mixture, but don't make it too sloppy. Shape the mixture into six to eight cakes.

Put seasoned flour in one bowl, beaten egg in another bowl and breadcrumbs in a third bowl. Dip each fish cake in flour, then egg and then breadcrumbs. Heat oil in a frying pan and fry until the fish cakes are golden brown on both sides.

Serve with some sweet chilli sauce.

Lean beef and lamb

Despite some concerns regarding the role of red meat as a possible risk factor in cancer development, it is important to know that in most of the studies on this there has been little distinction between the quality and type of red meat consumed. Lean lamb or beef, trimmed of all visible fat, makes an important contribution to a treatment diet. It offers high quality protein with all the essential amino acids required by the body; it is a key source of iron needed to help boost blood counts, as well as zinc, potassium and a range of B vitamins including thiamin, niacin and vitamins B6 and B12.

Like all red meats, lean high quality lamb or beef is most valued for its iron, which occurs as haem iron, the type most easily absorbed by the body. Iron is important for healthy blood, brain and immune function. It is somewhat perverse that people who usually eat red meat decide to cut this important food just as they are about to start their treatment, in which treatments like chemotherapy and radiotherapy affect blood – and if surgery is involved, there is often some blood loss and need for tissue repair and healing.

Also, lamb is particularly environmental as it is a grass feeder and accumulates fewer chemicals or toxins as it is killed when young. If you are having trouble with your taste buds, try some mint or fruity marinades.

Bread and pittas, rice and potatoes

One of my favourite food groups encompasses the healthy versions of bread, pittas and potatoes. Wholegrains are a nutrition power plant, while these foods also contain slow-releasing or lower GI type carbohydrates which help keep energy levels constant throughout the day. When portions are contained they are also a low-energy dense food which can be helpful if you are trying to control your weight.

Other examples of foods made with wholegrain or wholemeal ingredients include wholemeal and mixed-grain breads, rolls, wraps, flatbreads and English muffins, wholegrain breakfast cereals, wheat or oat flake breakfast biscuits, wholegrain crispbreads, rolled oats, wholemeal pasta, brown rice, popcorn, bulgar (cracked wheat) and rice cakes.

Wholegrains are low in fat and are important sources of protein, dietary fibre (lignans, beta-glucan and soluble pentosans), vitamins (especially B-group vitamins and antioxidant vitamin E), minerals (iron, zinc, magnesium and selenium) and many bioactive phyto-chemicals, including:

- phytosterols – which have cholesterol-lowering properties;
- sphingolipids – which are associated with tumour control and maintenance of normal epithelia;
- polyphenols and phenolics – such as hydroxycinnamic, ferulic, vanillic and p-coumaric acids, which have antioxidant properties;
- carotenoids – such as alpha- and beta-carotene, lutein and zeax-anthin, which have antioxidant functions;
- phytates – which may have a role in lowering glycaemic responses and reducing oxidation of cholesterol.

Antioxidants in wholegrains

The antioxidant content of wholegrains is worthy of note, with research showing that the *in vitro* antioxidant activity of whole-grain foods is on a par with, or higher than, that of vegetables and fruits. A 2007 study by the Agricultural Research Service of the United States Department of Agriculture ranked foods for their anti-oxidant capacity. Cereal-based foods including ready-to-eat cereals, oats, wholegrain breads and legumes were found to be among the highest antioxidant-containing foods by ORAC (oxygen radical absorbance capacity) score, as shown in Table 5.3.

As you can see, based on quantities consumed, in some cases grain foods provide higher amounts of antioxidants than most fruits and vegetables. The antioxidant vitamins in grains, such as vitamin E and its isomers (tocopherols and tocotrienols), and minerals such as selenium contribute to the antioxidant activity as phytochemicals like phytates, phenolics and lignans or alkylresorcinols.

There are also some grain-specific antioxidants, such as ory-zonol in rice, avenanthramides in oats and ferulic acid in corn and wheat. Certain other phenolics, phenolic lipids, flavonoids, tocopherols and dietary fibres (e.g. beta-glucan) found in grains are

Table 5.3 ORAC antioxidant capacity of selected fruits, vegetables, grains and legumes

Grains	Fruit and vegetables	Legumes
Rice bran 24,287	Blueberries 6,552	Pinto beans 904
Cornflakes 2,359	Blackberries 5,347	Carrots 666
Granola 2,294	Strawberries 3,577	Chickpeas 847
Oat bran 2,183	Apples 2,828	Green peas 600
Rolled oats 2,169	Avocados 1,933	Lima beans 243
Pumpernickel 1,963	Oranges 1,819	
Popcorn 1,743	Spinach 1,515	
Mixed grain bread 1,421	Broccoli 1,362	
Shredded Wheat cereal 1,303	Green tea, brewed 1,253	
	Mangoes 1,002	

anti-mutagenic and anti-inflammatory. This means they can help prevent cancer.

Choline, betaine and alkylresorcinols (particularly abundant in rye) are other important compounds found in wholegrains which play a role in the prevention of cell mutations (cell mistakes) and tumour formation.

Research has shown (and continues to bring to light) the many nutritional and functional components of wholegrain cereals that work alone and/or in synergy to promote good health and help reduce risks of certain types of cancer. I have also included some additional information on boosting antioxidant intakes across your diet in the fruits and vegetables recipes below.

Recipes

Popcorn snack

Popcorn is a great source of fibre and provides a big antioxidant boost. It is a great snack food that should not just be reserved for the movies. If you need to boost your weight the taste is enhanced with some melted butter and a little salt. Those on a stricter energy budget can enjoy it plain with just a sprinkle of salt for extra flavour.

Put ¼ cup raw corn kernels (I prefer the raw kernels to the pre-packaged microwave variety) into a large microwave dish. Put the lid on and then cook on high in the microwave for 2–3 minutes. Add butter or salt as desired.

Tuna and corn jacket potatoes

Try these tantalizingly tasty jacket potatoes.

4 large (1.2 kg) sebago potatoes (baby or new potatoes can be used if you would prefer to eat a lower GI potato)

425 g can tuna in spring water, drained and flaked

2 x 125 g cans corn kernels, drained and rinsed

¼ cup whole-egg mayonnaise

1 spring onion, thinly sliced diagonally

Position oven rack just above centre of oven. Preheat oven to 200° C/180° C fan/400° F/Gas Mark 6. Scrub and rinse potatoes. Pat dry. Pierce each potato six times with a fork and wrap in foil. Place on oven rack. Bake for 1 hour 30 minutes or until tender when a skewer is inserted into centre. Transfer to a plate. Stand for 10 minutes.

Combine tuna, corn and mayonnaise in a bowl. Season with salt and pepper. Remove foil from potatoes and cut a deep cross in the top of each. Using a tea towel to protect your hands, take each one and squeeze the base gently to open the top. Place potatoes on plates and top with tuna mixture and a sprinkling of onion. Serves four.

Darker coloured fruits and vegetables

Fruits and vegetables are an essential part of a treatment diet plan, as they provide the body with many essential nutrients including vitamins, minerals and the phytochemicals. The most benefit comes from eating as many different varieties as you can, and generally the darker and richer the colour, the higher the level of these phytochemicals. This means throwing extra dark green leafy vegetables into pasta dishes, stews, omelettes and so on – my kids never notice when I put grated courgette (zucchini) in their brownies! Red fruits such as frozen berries work well in crumbles and smoothies and mixed with meringues.

Here are some other ways to boost your intake of fruit and vegetables:

- Add some fresh fruit or dried fruit to your cereal in the morning, e.g. sultanas and banana go well on porridge, as does a handful of blueberries.
- Include a piece of fresh fruit as a morning or afternoon snack. A banana is easy to grab as you are walking out of the door, and remember to put a couple of pieces of fruit in your bag before you leave home. It's also an idea to keep some dried fruit in the car or in your bag. I suggest the organic apricots which are dark in colour.
- Always add lots of salad to your sandwich or have a salad at lunch. This is easy with ready-prepared bags of leafy green salad. A handful of rocket gives a fresh, peppery taste to any salad or sandwich.
- Enjoy a hot cup of vegetable soup for lunch or as a snack. If you are unable to prepare these yourself, try out some of the supermarket options. There are some lovely varieties of soups in the chill section and the old canned soups can work just as well.
- Fill your plate with at least two or three colours of vegetables in the evening. If you are not eating as well as you normally do, then you can fork-mash these or blend them. (Puréed carrot and swede with butter is particularly nice, maybe with a teaspoon of sugar and a squeeze of lemon juice.)
- Keep some frozen or canned fruit in the cupboard to add to recipes or puddings (e.g. tinned peaches or apricots in lime jelly).
- Visit the local markets to pick up some seasonal fruit and vegetables, or organize a regular delivery of a seasonal box.
- Adapt your recipes to include more vegetables or fruit. For example, bolognese sauce is good with grated carrot, courgettes, aubergines and a small can of kidney beans. Add extra vegetables such as peas, carrots and swede to stews. Try something different, like a vegetarian curry, and add chickpeas.
- Grill some Mediterranean vegetables like red and green peppers, aubergines, asparagus and artichokes, and drizzle with a little olive oil (a good way to boost the energy content of your food).
- Dry-roast a selection of starchy vegetables such as sweet potato, parsnip, butternut squash, swede, celeriac, etc.

- Include lots of the brassica family of vegetables, such as broccoli, cauliflower, cabbage or brussels sprouts. However, if your treatment is causing bowel problems it may be best to limit these foods.

Herbs and spices

Although herbs and spices have long been a part of our history, most of us do not use them anywhere near enough. Not only do herbs and spices impart a wide range of flavours, aromas and textures to foods – which is very useful if the taste buds need a bit of a kick – but they are in fact the most concentrated sources of antioxidants and other phytochemicals.

One which has been in the spotlight is curcumin, the active component of turmeric. It is a powerful antioxidant with a similar potency to vitamins C and E. It also has wide-ranging effects on the body's immune system, acting on lymphocytes and other immune cells as well as enhancing wound-healing. Additionally some studies have found that curcumin can help prevent tumour growth, kill cancerous cells, arrest the spread of cancer and disrupt the tumour's blood supply. Turmeric is a very versatile flavour which works well in a mild chicken curry, sprinkled on roasted vegetables or added to soups. When it is mixed with a little oil and black pepper, the potent nutrients are absorbed over a thousand times better than if taken in a capsule form.

Chicken curry

Try this simple but delicious turmeric-containing chicken curry recipe. Minced chicken can also be used if a softer texture is needed.

2 tablespoons vegetable oil
2 large chicken breast fillets, skinned and cut into chunks
1 clove garlic, finely chopped
1 large onion, sliced and chopped
½ teaspoon ground ginger
½ teaspoon chilli powder (optional and best left out if the mouth is a little raw)

½ teaspoon ground cinnamon
½ teaspoon ground turmeric
½ teaspoon ground white pepper
250 g tinned chopped tomatoes
4 tablespoons chicken stock
2 tablespoon ground almonds
4 tablespoons double cream
4 tablespoons plain yoghurt

Heat oil in a frying pan and fry chicken, garlic and onion until chicken is cooked through (cut open a small piece to test that it is no longer pink). Season with ginger, chilli powder, cinnamon, turmeric and white pepper and set the heat to medium. Mix in the tomatoes and chicken stock. Return to a simmer, and then stir in the almonds. Stir in cream and yoghurt, and then cook gently for 2 to 4 minutes, before serving on a bed of rice. Serves four.

Ginger is another helpful spice as it also may offer a range of anti-cancer and therapeutic properties. There are at least 50 antioxidants from the rhizome of ginger. One of these, the active component gingerol, has suppressed tumour growth and tumour blood supply and killed cancerous cells in several human lab experiments. Ginger is also known for its anti-nausea properties.

The key to harnessing the benefits from herbs and spices is to use them in their whole form, added to food, rather than taking a supplement form. Herbs and spices are also great to give a health

Table 5.4 Herbs and spices

Herbs and spices	Activity	Flavour	Uses
Anise	Reportedly can help boost appetite and inhibit cancer-stimulating enzymes	Warm minty/liquorice taste	
Basil	A beneficial antioxidant, and reported to have digestive properties	Spicy, minty flavour	Great with tomatoes, lemons, fish, chicken, pasta, pizza, salads, dressings and teas Best added at the end of cooking
Black pepper	Enhances antioxidant enzymes	Spicy flavour that enhances natural flavours of food	Can be added to all savoury dishes

(continued)

Table 5.4 *continued*

Herbs and spices	Activity	Flavour	Uses
Cloves	Highest concentration of polyphenol antioxidants	Spicy, fruity flavour	Great added to fruit dishes such as apple crumbles and pies, and goes well with nutmeg-type dishes
Fennel	Reported as a digestive aid	Sweet, liquorice flavour	Lovely over salads, fish such as salmon, soup and cooked vegetables Can also be added to mashed potato
Garlic	High in many minerals including magnesium, zinc, sodium and potassium Source of Vitamins A, B and C Contains some potent antioxidants	A strong flavour, use sparingly	A must with tomato- and onion-based dishes, roasted meats and pesto, and great in stews and soups Try adding roasted varieties with salad dressing and roasted vegetables, or making some garlic bread, squeezing out the flesh for a more gentle, creamy flavour
Rosemary	Antioxidant and antibacterial properties	Can vary from eucalyptus to pine-like	Awesome with lamb, roasted vegetables, fish and soups, and in bread
Mint	Reported as a digestive aid and has antioxidant properties	Mint flavour	Makes a refreshing cup of tea Great with yoghurt or vegetables and can be scattered over berries, served with cheese, other fruits and with lamb

This is just a starter list and I would recommend Jekka McVicar's book (see Further reading, p. 155) for further ideas on the tastes and use of the vast array of herbs and spices in cooking.

boost for individuals who are not managing to eat quite the variety of foods that they might normally have. They can be added to all textures of food, and spices like ginger, cinnamon and nutmeg can be added to smoothies and milk drinks.

Some of the other herbs and spices that you can try to incorporate in food and cooking are shown in Table 5.4.

Cooking to retain the nutrients in your fruits and vegetables

Many of the nutrients found in fruit and vegetables are highly unstable and easily destroyed by exposure to the environment (light, oxygen, soaking in water, heat). It is therefore better to prepare fruit and vegetables in a way that retains most of their nutritional value.

- Try eating vegetables raw whenever possible, e.g. cut up crudités or grated cabbage in salads or coleslaw. This is a good snack for both you and the kids before dinner.
- Try to use fruit and vegetables when fresh. Keep in the fridge until needed.
- Cut into large chunks rather than little bits.
- Steam or microwave vegetables in small amounts of water rather than boiling with lots of water. If possible, re-use the water in your cooking as an addition to a sauce or gravy.
- Avoid unnecessary peeling or slicing and try to keep the skins on vegetables like potato, sweet potato and tomatoes to increase the fibre content.

6

Coping with side effects: nausea and vomiting, taste changes and fatigue

I do my best to reassure people I meet that while it may seem overwhelming to hear about all the unpleasant side effects, the intention of providing this detail at the outset is simply to be prepared. Forewarned is forearmed. *But* do bear in mind that it is hard to predict exactly how each individual will react to particular treatments. So while it is good to understand potential side effects, before I let you go on to explore the ideas and Food Fix suggestions in this chapter, I do ask you please not to panic. I do not want you to feel overwhelmed, or to wonder why you are going through all this – though, understandably, almost everyone does at some stage.

First, not everyone experiences difficult side effects during treatment, and even in cases where side effects do have a debilitating impact, help is available. This is a time when, more than ever, you will be closely monitored and supported by your doctor and the clinical team. So, in addition to my Food Fix suggestions, your healthcare team will arm you with many more strategies including medications to help you get through. Many clinics now also employ a range of support services such as aromatherapy, which many people find useful.

Using food to combat side effects

This is where the idea of adjusting your normal eating habits, discussed in earlier chapters, really comes into play. It means being flexible and creative, and adapting your normal dietary approach to whatever gets the calories and nutrients in. As I always say, it's a time when you need to tune into your body and recognize that while the anti-cancer diet books might give more ticks to the super-green salad, you and your body might find it easier to sip on some cola and nibble on a packet of salty crisps. Now is when you put on your Heston Blumenthal/celebrity chef hat and experiment with new tastes that might include extra, fewer or new flavours, a range of textures which could have a crunch or be silky smooth, food temperatures from cold to hot, and even when you schedule your eating. Some people feel better in the morning and should take more food then, while others need to take a mouthful every hour, and still others feel better later in the day.

I always remember, early in my career, working with a gentleman who had lost his sense of taste but found that he could pick up the flavour of soy sauce – and so he ended up putting soy sauce on just about everything he ate. This was right through from his breakfast cereal to his ice cream! While to you and me this might sound absolutely disgusting, it is a perfect example of creatively reframing your normal food likes and doing whatever works.

Most experienced cancer dietitians have a big bag of tricks that they can pull out to help deal with side effects. This is in conjunction with the clinical team, who can arm you with many very effective medications that reduce or prevent these side effects. Here I must quickly add that if you are asked to take something to prevent nausea or to help your bowels work properly, you should stick to the regime you have been given. I have lost count of the number of times I have questioned someone who has been losing weight because of nausea, asking what drug has been prescribed and when it is supposed to be taken, only to be told, 'I didn't want to take any extra medicines and wanted to try to fight these symptoms on my own.' Of course, if you have any concerns about specific medications or if you have noticed that they contribute to other unpleasant side effects, these should be discussed with your doctor or pharmacist, but this is definitely not the time to take a high and mighty approach to dealing with side effects. Many of these symptoms, such as nausea, can be debilitating and unlike a headache, for example, don't always just go away.

So this is the know-how chapter that gives you practical strategies to help you get through any challenges with the best possible outcome. This chapter has been set out to allow you to go straight to the topics that are relevant to you. The idea is that you can flick back and forth as need be while you experiment with your diet to help *you* do your best to counter the impact that a poor dietary intake can have. The reason I highlight 'you' is to gently remind you that the doctors and nurses are working hard to kill off or at least control your cancer, but only *you* can invest in the effort to prevent drastic weight losses and the associated issues of suboptimal nutritional intake.

Whatever happens, I want you to take seriously the need to eat well in the context of cancer and its treatment, even – and especially – when it goes against previously acceptable thinking about 'losing weight'.

I know that it is just so hard for some individuals to imagine ever losing their appetite, or having food not taste the same way, or possibly losing large amounts of weight. As most have had the opposite problem with weight gain, I know that many people in the early stages think that the weight loss is quite positive, and when I am talking to them about boosting their intake they often say, quite happily, 'I actually like being a stone or two lighter and I do not want to gain weight.' What they don't realize is that if they do not address their reduced food intake, that one stone quickly becomes two and then three, and that dress they want to fit into will fall off them. Many people turn to big overcoats or baggy jumpers (as they will also be feeling the cold) to cover up, as they dread the sight of their skeletal frame and do not want their friends or family to see it. They find their shape quite distressing and a horrible reminder of the illness they are dealing with.

I cannot stress enough the importance of not letting vanity get in the way. When it seems easier to miss a meal or play around with the food on the plate, you must try to do everything in your power to eat as normally as you can, and to find a way to take in the maximum amount of nutrients you need to help your body stay strong and keep your weight not too far away from where it normally is. It is almost impossible for individuals who end up becoming extremely wasted to rebuild the muscle lost during this treatment phase.

To do all this you will need to keep coming back to re-read sections of this book which may not have been relevant early on.

If despite your best efforts you are not managing with food or supplement drinks, then alternative options can be tried, such as feeding a formula through a tube into your stomach or further down the gut; this is known as enteral feeding. Very occasionally food nutrients have be infused through a drip directly into the bloodstream, a technique known as parenteral nutrition.

If alternative methods of feeding do need to be employed, try not to regard them as the end of the world. When I suggest enteral feeding, people often look at me as if I have told them that I have found another cancer in their body. It's understandable that people dread the prospect. However, the recommendation will be because they are likely to have (or are already having) such a terrible time trying to eat or take in liquids because of the impact of their treatment, such as surgery or other more intensive types of treatment. This means that the process of eating is either not possible or dangerous, or that it is going to be living hell for them. Once I sit down and explain how it all works and that there are amazing and dedicated home enteral feeding support services which are on call to back them up, the blood does come back to people's faces.

Drip or bolus feeding into the gut is always used as the first port of call if eating is not possible, rather than what might seem a more palatable option, feeding through a drip into a large vein. This is because the gut performs at its best when the nutrients pass through in a more normal way. The possible risks and complications associated with this type of feeding are much lower than those associated with what is called parenteral nutrition.

Nausea and vomiting

There can be nothing worse than trying to face food when you are feeling sick or have been bringing up your food. Persistent nausea has a debilitating effect on your food intake and quality of life. There are many reasons for nausea and vomiting and if you are experiencing problems you should discuss them with your doctor or clinic specialist immediately. This is especially if the vomiting continues, as there is the potential for you to become dehydrated quite quickly.

Fortunately nausea is not quite as a debilitating a problem as it used to be. This is because there is now a wider and more potent range of medications (anti-nausea drugs or anti-emetics). It is important to take the medication prescribed, preferably before rather than after you start to feel nauseous. This is something I really must emphasize. Many people take the view that it is better to try to fight their symptoms until they pass, instead of taking the pills they have been prescribed. I can't tell you how many times I have had to remind individuals to take these pills, even though they have been told to do so by their doctor and their clinical support team. If you are taking anti-emetic pills and are still experiencing problems, it is also important to contact your doctor or the clinical team. Again, there are so many new and stronger options around that can be tried.

Many people also find that therapies such as music, distraction, relaxation, aromatherapy and acupuncture help. They are all worth exploring.

One of the most effective dietary options is to try to take extra amounts of protein throughout the day. Research has shown that many people experience less nausea, especially delayed nausea or nausea after chemotherapy has ended, by sipping slowly on high protein (whey) drinks with powdered ginger twice a day.

The other important strategy, although it may seem counter-intuitive at a time when the sight and smell of food may make you feel unwell, is to eat or nibble on several small snacks, rather than larger meals.

Nausea is worse on an empty stomach. If you can't manage even small meals, just try to keep nibbling small amounts of food or sipping on sugar-containing drinks. I often suggest keeping a couple of dry water biscuits on the bedside table to nibble on before getting out of bed. Having something to line the stomach seems to help you to do better at breakfast.

Other nibble ideas can include crackers, cheese, cold hard-boiled eggs, rice pudding, nuts, olives, salty broth and soups, ginger beer, ginger biscuits, crystalline ginger, salt and vinegar crisps, cola, toast and Marmite or Vegemite.

Food Fix – tips for coping with nausea

- Try and ensure you're relaxed and comfortable when you eat, and that the room is quiet and airy. Sit to eat, don't stand or lie down.
- Stay away from hot, stuffy kitchens or canteens full of cooking odours. Also avoid pungent foods, such as fried food, fish, onions, garlic and curry or other spicy dishes.

- Eat a little of what you fancy – don't force yourself to eat, or eat foods out of duty or just because they're 'good for you'. Again, it might be easier to nibble on a dry cracker or some crisps or to sip cola (it works) instead of trying to be a purist who has made a pact with him- or herself to eat only fish and greens.
- Eat slowly, and chew the food properly.
- Check with your doctor about whether nausea medication should be taken before or with food.
- Keep a diary of when you feel sick or vomit while having treatment, and discuss this with your doctor.
- Try to catch up on your calories at times of the day when you feel better.
- Try and eat regularly, having meals and snacks at the same times each day.
- Make meals enjoyable social occasions when you can. Make time to chat with the family, lay the table with a cloth, add a vase of flowers and some candles.
- Avoid foods that are hot, greasy, fried, spicy, fatty or high in sugar. Eat foods that are cooler or at room temperature such as crackers and cheese, quiche, cold meat platters, olives, dips, crackers, nuts.
- Avoid alcohol and tobacco.
- Keep some salty crackers or pretzels beside your bed for when you wake up.
- Reheat meals in the oven instead of the microwave.
- Sip on fluids like lemon-flavoured barley water, broth or clear juice, or suck ice lollies. Try refreshing fluids like elderflower cordial or jelly or the ginger squash recipe on page 79.
- You can also try sucking on ice, made either of plain water or frozen fruit juice. Avoid drinking too much fluid with meals, as this can make you feel full and bloated.
- If you can't eat solid foods, try liquid meal replacements.
- Keep your mouth fresh, and if there is an unpleasant taste, suck on peppermints.
- Stick to light, plain foods on treatment days like chicken soup (see recipe on page 79) or rice pudding.
- If you can, eat nutritious, high protein snacks such as peanut butter and crackers, cheese and crackers or nuts. Otherwise, try plain bland foods, such as plain crackers, toast, dry cereals, plain yogurt, etc.

- Try a Sea-Band, a wristband that some find can help control nausea.
- If the nausea continues, try having a rest and then see if you can nibble on something light when you wake.

Table 6.1 has some more ideas on how to get through a day when you are feeling nauseated.

Table 6.1 Getting through a day when you feel nauseous

Before getting out of bed	Eat a water biscuit or salty wheat cracker, or take a handful of almonds.
Breakfast	Take a slice of white toast with a thin spread of butter and a salty spread such as Marmite or Vegemite, or a higher protein food such as a slice of cheese, an egg or some nut butter. If this is too much, stick with the salty crackers, either plain or with a salty or high protein spread.
Morning snack	Sip slowly on ginger beer (use a straw) or try Coca-Cola or ginger squash (see recipe on page 79). Nibble on nuts, ginger biscuits or crackers or pretzels. Try a chilled whey protein supplement drink (use a straw).
Lunch	Try a lean piece of chicken breast, a quality slice of ham or a boiled egg, or some turkey breast with soft white bread and butter (lean, high protein foods are recommended). Add a little extra salt.
Afternoon snack	Try rice pudding, tinned peaches or pears, jelly, ice lollies or custard, or stick to the salty nibbles like pretzels, salted or flavoured rice cakes, or a piece of white bread or toast with a salty spread like Marmite or a piece of cheddar cheese. Try a chilled whey protein supplement drink (use a straw).
Small evening meal or snack	Try the homemade chicken soup recipe on page 79 or any broth-type recipe. If possible, try to include some chopped chicken or turkey added to the soup. Try a boiled egg with toast or an omelette with bacon (try to have someone else prepare this for you). A toasted sandwich may suit – try cheese, ham or some turkey.
Evening snack	You may also do better with a high protein sip feed or you can try to prepare your own versions, adding one of the high protein supplements to either a milk- or juice-based drink.

Some recipes to help you if you are struggling with nausea

Refreshing ginger squash

1 lime
7 cm piece fresh ginger, peeled and
   sliced crossways

⅓ cup caster sugar
Chilled or warm tea or soda water
   to serve

Peel the rind from the lime and then juice the lime flesh. Place sugar, ginger, lime rind, lime juice and 1.5 litres of water in a saucepan. Stir over a low heat until the sugar dissolves. Bring to the boil, reduce heat to medium–low and simmer for 10 minutes. Set aside to cool. Strain and store in a jug in the fridge.

To serve, add as a squash to either warm or cold tea or soda water and ice.

Chicken soup

This soup is easy, and the combination flavour of lemon and soy sauce works well.

Small chicken or chicken pieces
   (1.4 kg)
2 large onions, finely chopped
2 cups loosely packed fresh
   continental parsley leaves
¼ cup fresh lemon juice (extra
   can be added if a more intense
   lemon flavour is desired)

4 cloves garlic, crushed
2 tablespoons soy sauce (extra can
   be added)
5 medium carrots, cut into 1 cm
   pieces
2 medium tomatoes
Salt and pepper to taste
1.5 litres of water

If using a whole chicken, remove as much of the skin and the fat as possible. Combine the onions, parsley, garlic, lemon juice and soy sauce in a large saucepan and cook over a medium to low heat for 5–8 minutes or until the onions are soft (be careful not to burn them). Add chicken, celery, carrots and tomatoes and season with salt and pepper if taste buds need it, otherwise add some more chopped parsley. Add the water and bring to the boil. Reduce heat to low and simmer covered for 1 hour or until the chicken is tender and comes away from the bone easily. Remove from heat, stand for 10 minutes and place the soup in the fridge to chill overnight. (This allows the fat to rise to surface and set).

When ready to serve, remove the soup from the fridge and use a large metal spoon to remove the layer of solidified fat from the surface. Then remove the chicken from the soup and place in a large bowl. Pick the meat off the bones and shred into pieces. Discard the bones and return the meat to the soup. Bring the soup to the boil over a medium heat and simmer until the chicken and vegetables are heated through. Remove the soup from the heat and skim a piece of paper towel over the surface to absorb any excess fat. Season with salt and pepper as needed and serve in soup bowls with a piece of crusty bread.

Put single servings of the soup into storage containers and freeze, ready for when you need your next home-made chicken soup fix.

Fruity protein shake

300 ml apple juice (or use pineapple/other flavours blend)
1 scoop ice cream
½ large banana (optional)

4 frozen strawberries
2 scoops vanilla whey protein powder (available online or from health food stores)

Blend all ingredients together using a hand-held blender.

Chocolate coffee shake

2 scoops of chocolate protein powder or other protein
1 cup skimmed milk

5 ice cubes
1 cup water
1 teaspoon instant coffee granules

Blend all ingredients together using a hand-held blender.

Stomach soother

1 cup orange juice
¼ cup lemon juice

1 tablespoon corn syrup or honey
1 pint crushed ice

Mix the first three ingredients and pour on to the crushed ice. Take a small sip every 5–10 minutes.

Note: corn syrup can be replaced with glucose syrup or made up using the following substitutions: ½ cup sugar + 2 tbsp water = ½ cup light corn syrup; ½ cup honey = ½ cup light corn syrup.

Taste changes

Losing your sense of taste or experiencing strange or unpleasant flavours in your mouth, such as metallic, salty or sour flavours, is one of the most difficult-to-manage side effects of certain types of chemotherapy and radiotherapy. It is also an area where more research is needed. Unlike most other side effects, there are no medications available to help restore the taste buds. This means it is up to you to work out what tastes or flavours you can register and then start to get a bit wild or perhaps a bit weird with flavour mixtures, going to town with extra flavour additions such as sugar, salt, herbs, tomato ketchup, soy sauce, honey, apple juice, pineapple juice, elderflower cordial, vanilla milky flavours, mint, garlic, coriander, basil, etc.

You need to work out what concoctions or mixtures of flavours to incorporate into your food so that you can at least register something. If you have completely lost your sense of taste it is important to use lots of colours, different textures (crunch or smooth) and various temperatures to help keep your food interesting and manageable. Keeping your mouth clean and fresh is also a must.

At times, low zinc levels can cause problems with taste acuity. So if you have lost your sense of taste after not having eaten well for a period of time it is worth discussing with your doctor whether to have your zinc levels screened.

Experiment with the following Food Fix ideas for taste changes.

Food Fix – tips for coping with taste changes

- If your taste buds are not responding to the flavours you normally enjoy, adjust both flavours and textures (i.e. smooth or crunchy) to find alternatives that can work for you at the moment.
- Foods that are strong in flavour may be preferred – choose stronger flavours of enjoyed foods like a stronger cheese, Asian sauces or marinades, Lebanese spices like harissa, preserved lemons.
- Sauces, seasonings, gravy, herbs, marinades, pickles and spices can all help to add extra taste.
- Experiment with different foods and tastes, or if there is no taste add crunch or other textures like smooth, minced or fizz (try flavoured mineral waters).

- Avoid very cold or hot foods.
- If meat tastes bitter, try soaking it in wine, soy sauce or fruit juices. Also try avoiding foods sweetened with saccharine, which may exacerbate this.
- Clearing the palate with a glass of water and lemon juice before eating can help to enhance taste.
- Take refreshing drinks such as herbal teas, orange juice or lemonade.
- Keep the mouth and teeth clean.
- Rinse or brush teeth before eating.
- Use toothpaste that is non-mint flavour – this may help to reduce aberrant tastes in the mouth.
- Try using a spray mister before and during meals.
- If a metallic taste is present, try using plastic or glass utensils.
- If a metallic or bitter taste is present, try sucking on sugar-free mints, lemon drops or chewing gum.
- Avoid favourite foods and drinks altogether while taste changes persist – this helps to stop you developing a dislike for them in the long term.
- Avoid the foods that taste strange but re-try every few weeks, as your sense of taste may have changed back to normal. The most common foods affected by changes in taste are citrus fruits, chocolate, tea and red meats.
- Often the sweet tastes are the first to return and so it is worth trying more sweet marinades, honey, brown sugar and other sweet flavours. Meat is often better if it is marinated in a sweet or Asian type sauce.

Here are some examples of flavour mixes to try with food.

Roasted tomato and basil soup

8–10 medium-sized ripe tomatoes, seeded and cut into quarters

1 large sweet red pepper, cut into large chunks

2 x 425 g cans organic diced tomatoes, including juice

2 medium yellow onions, chopped

4 cups chicken or vegetable broth (I use Massel)

1 cup firmly packed finely chopped fresh basil leaves

½ cup sun-dried tomatoes or ½ cup Heinz tomato soup (a flavour many people crave)

¼ cup cold-pressed extra-virgin olive oil

8 large cloves fresh garlic, finely chopped

¼ cup raw macadamia nuts (optional)

2 teasp fresh thyme leaves (lemon thyme if available)

2 teasp sea salt

Freshly ground black pepper to taste

Olive oil for frying

Preheat oven to 200° C/180° C fan/400° F/Gas Mark 6. Toss together the sweet pepper, fresh tomato quarters, olive oil, 1 teaspoon of the salt and a sprinkle of cracked pepper. Spread in a single layer on a baking sheet and roast for about an hour, giving everything a good toss a couple of times during the cooking to get an even roast.

In a large pot, sauté the onions and garlic in a couple of tablespoons of olive oil with the remaining salt for about 10 minutes until the onions just start to brown. Add the canned tomatoes with all of their juices, the basil, thyme and chicken or vegetable broth, together with the oven-roasted pepper and tomatoes with all of their juices and the sun-dried tomatoes. Bring this mixture to a boil and simmer uncovered for about 30 minutes.

Place the mixture in your blender in batches with the macadamias and blend until smooth and creamy. Season to taste and serve with crusty bread or a scoop of your favourite grain. For extra protein and to turn it into a meal, you can add some cooked, shredded chicken. Serves six to eight.

Experiment with the seasoning and flavours. Some people need two or three times more than usual to hit the spot.

Chai tea – an Indian tea with milk and spices

10 green cardamom pods, cracked, seeds removed and pods discarded, or ½ teaspoon cardamom seeds or ground cardamom

4 cm piece cinnamon stick

4 peppercorns (preferably white)

¼ teaspoon fennel seeds

2 cups whole milk (use high protein milk)

3½ tablespoons packed light brown sugar, or to taste

½ teaspoon ground ginger

Pinch salt

2 cups water

5 teaspoons loose orange pekoe tea or other black tea

You will also need a mortar and pestle or an electric coffee or spice grinder

Grind together the cardamom, cinnamon stick, peppercorns and fennel seeds with a mortar and pestle or coffee/spice grinder.

Bring milk just to a simmer in a 2-litre heavy saucepan. Stir or whisk in brown sugar, ground spice mixture, ginger and a little salt to taste. Reduce heat to low and simmer gently, stirring occasionally, for 3 minutes to infuse the flavours.

Meanwhile, bring the water to a boil in a 1-litre saucepan, add the tea and boil for 1 minute. Pour through a fine-mesh sieve into hot milk mixture (discard tea leaves) and cook over low heat for 1 minute. Stir before serving.

Chai tea can be also purchased at Starbucks or in the tea section of supermarkets. Shop around to find a brand that best suits your tastes.

Guacamole

2 avocados, peeled, stones
   removed, flesh roughly chopped
4 spring onions, thinly sliced
1 tomato, finely diced

¼ cup coriander leaves, finely
   chopped
1 lime, juiced
Salt and pepper

Place avocados in a shallow dish and mash with a fork until smooth. Add onions, tomato, coriander, 2 tablespoons lime juice and salt and pepper. Stir until well combined. Cover surface with plastic wrap. Refrigerate until ready to serve.

Guacamole will keep, covered, in the fridge for up to three days. For a creamier taste that is higher in energy, add ¼ cup sour cream. Experiment with the amount of lime and coriander flavours.

Mexican flavour mix

Made with chilli powder and toasted cumin seeds, this gives an authentic kick to Mexican favourites, such as tacos and burritos. Once prepared it can be added to mince or chicken. If your mouth is raw you may need to limit or avoid chilli powder.

1 tablespoon cumin seeds
1 tablespoon dried coriander leaves
1 tablespoon mild paprika

1 teaspoon ground oregano
½ teaspoon chilli powder
½ teaspoon garlic powder

Place cumin in a non-stick frying pan over medium heat. Cook, stirring, for 1–2 minutes or until aromatic. Transfer to a mortar. Gently pound with a pestle until coarsely crushed.

Stir in the coriander, paprika, oregano, chilli powder and garlic powder.

To use, combine the spice mix with mashed avocado, sour cream and lemon juice. Serve with corn chips for dipping. Or for Mexican beef tacos, add to mince mixture, divide among taco shells and top with salsa, chopped avocado and grated cheddar to serve.

Fatigue

Fatigue is an all too common symptom of cancer and tends to be the symptom that troubles people most. On average, 80 per cent of people with cancer experience tiredness, often of a deep, debilitating kind. This kind of fatigue is often made worse if you are not eating enough or if you are not eating the right foods, and presents yet another reason why it's so important to make the effort to eat properly. Sometimes even a very small meal of the right kind, nicely presented and enjoyed, can make a noticeable difference to how you feel, and give you that little bit more energy to keep going.

Reasons for fatigue are complex and may include waste products of tumour breakdown and increased nutritional demands. Additional factors can include anaemia, inadequate food intake, decreased activity and poor sleep. Fatigue can also be due to dehydration.

Food Fix – tips for coping with fatigue

To help manage the chores of shopping and food preparation, you may need to juggle your usual routine a little, making the most of the times when you have more energy.

Use a fatigue diary to monitor times when you feel better and to highlight any particular activities that increase the fatigue. Then plan your shopping and cooking around this. Make the most of the not-so-tired time by doing the shopping in the morning when the supermarket may be quieter. Internet shopping is another option – keep lists of basics from week to week to save time and trouble. I also suggest that you play around with the different supermarket websites, as many of them include a recipe section which allows you to choose some new dishes that might suit you, with the option of adding the ingredients to your shopping basket. I also encourage you to get friends and family to help organize the shopping and freezer stocks. And enjoy the cooking – sit down to prepare food, listen to some music, and generally take it easy.

- When you are feeling more energetic, prepare a few bulk recipes such as bolognese sauces, lasagnes, meat- or chicken-based soups, stews and curries to put into individual freezer bags. Incorporating more meals with lean protein foods including red meat can also help boost iron and blood counts, which may be one cause of the fatigue.

- Invest in a few good quality readymade meals for the freezer. Some of these can be rather salty but you can mitigate this by adding extra vegetables, such as a handful of frozen peas. Look for quality supermarket brands. Wiltshire Farm Foods (<http://www.wiltshirefarmfoods.com>) offer a range of delicious meals, including a modified textured or special diet range, which can be ordered over the phone or internet.

- Keep a good supply of tins so that you have the ingredients to hand for very simple, easy-to-prepare meals such as baked beans or sardines on toast, or a hearty bean-based soup. Other tins worth having include tuna, beans and pulses, vegetables such as mini-carrots, artichokes or asparagus, and fruit such as apricots, prunes or raspberries. Tinned tomatoes make a great sauce for a range of pasta dishes; tinned salmon can make tastier fishcakes than fresh salmon. Try tinned potatoes gently sautéed in butter or olive oil. Tinned Irish stew boosts your protein and iron intake, and you can add vitamins with extra home-cooked vegetables. Tinned rice pudding can be delicious, especially if you add a scrap of lemon rind and a sprinkling of nutmeg, and maybe a stirring of cream too – and it boosts your calcium levels.

- Make use of local delicatessens, farmers' markets or food shops for treats – some speciality bread baked on the premises, perhaps, with a few shavings of good quality ham and a few olives.

- Go out for a local meal if you do not feel like cooking. Often getting out of the house and enjoying something different can give you a lift.

- Keep handy the numbers of local takeaways or restaurants that deliver to your door.

- Have some desserts like custard or yoghurt in the fridge, some powdered or UHT milk in case you run out of regular milk, dried, tinned or frozen fruit, portion packs of cheese and cereal bars, nut mixes – all these are helpful to have on hand to keep energy topped up if you are out attending appointments. It is important to snack regularly to help keep your energy levels up; missing your meals will only drain your reserves further.

Some recipes to help you out if you are struggling with fatigue

Food for fatigue has to be all about ease and convenience. It is also important to be flexible and to use a few more convenience meals and snacks. Once upon a time I would never have picked up a frozen or chilled meal from a supermarket, but these days, in response to the demands of consumers, the stores have worked hard to improve the taste, quality and nutritional standards of these meals. If you haven't been near this section of the supermarket for some time it is worth a revisit.

The food you eat at this time needs to be easy to eat and enticing and should serve to help pick you up. This means a dish should look and taste appetizing, use a few more special or better quality ingredients and slide down easily rather than requiring too much chewing. You may do better with a mornay that includes some delicious fresh salmon mixed in with some pasta than trying to chomp your way through a big piece of steak.

Easy creamy chicken pasta

Drizzle of olive oil
1 onion, chopped
500 g chicken thigh fillets
375 ml tin Carnation Evaporated Milk Light
45 g packet chicken noodle soup mix

1 teaspoon minced garlic
2 teaspoons cornflour mixed with a little cold water (to thicken, if needed)
Pasta (shells or penne or bows but it doesn't matter)

Cook onion in oil until translucent. Add chicken pieces and stir through. Sprinkle soup mix over chicken, add Evaporated Milk and simmer while pasta cooks. (Cream cheese works well as a substitute for the evaporated milk.) Cook pasta until al dente; drain. Thicken sauce with the cornflour mixture if necessary. Add sauce to pasta, mix thoroughly and serve. Serves four.

Slow cooker

If you have a slow cooker it is ideal for easy meals – such as the following:

Easy beef stroganoff

Sliced rump steak	1 teaspoon cornflour
A little seasoned flour	Mushrooms, sliced
2 tablespoons tomato paste	1–2 cloves garlic
2 cups of chicken or beef stock	Sour cream (or light option)

Slow cooker: roll the sliced steak in seasoned flour. Place all ingredients except sour cream into slow cooker. Cook on the auto setting until steak is tender and cooked through, 4–5 hours.

Oven: preheat oven to 180° C/160° C fan/350° F/Gas Mark 4. Prepare as above and cook for about 1 hour, stirring occasionally.

Frying pan: cook steak and onion. Add chicken stock, tomato paste, mushrooms and garlic and simmer for about 15 minutes.

All methods: when cooked, stir in the sour cream and added sifted cornflour to thicken. Serve with pasta.

This was one of my mother's family recipes and it highlights the use of timesaving utensils for cooking. Many people find a slow cooker a worthwhile investment. It allows you to do more of the food preparation earlier in the day and return home to a lovely delicious meal that is ready to go. I certainly know puddings work very well too.

Your local library or bookstore may have books of slow cooker recipes – or there's a wide range of recipes online (see <http://southernfood.about.com/library/crock/blcpidx.htm> or <http://allrecipes.co.uk/recipes/slow-cooker-recipes.aspx>).

7

Coping with side effects: others (pre- and post-surgery, constipation, diarrhoea, etc.)

Ensuring you are nutritionally strong and well prepared for surgery is very important. Some surgeons support the need to spend a few weeks building up the nutrition stores before an operation, and if it is a major operation they may recommend special nutritional formula drinks designed to help improve response and recovery times.

While the impact of surgery on nutrition depends on where and what type of surgery you are undergoing, the body will repair and recover at a faster rate if the higher protein and nutrient requirements can be provided for. This would mean a protein intake of around 1.8–2.0 g per kilogram of body weight.

Some of the compounding problems around nutritional health at this time may include whether the tumour has affected dietary intake before the surgery (for example, a tumour might have made swallowing difficult), the anxiety around the surgery, the hospital food, the impact of the operation itself and the expected length of the recovery period.

Quite often there are lengthy periods of nil by mouth, both for tests and for the operation itself, and if your surgery involves the gut it can take some time before you are able to tolerate a normal diet.

After surgery you might need to test the water by starting on clear fluids (apple juice, jelly, black tea), the free fluids (milk, yoghurt, custard) and soft food (mashed potato, puréed apple), and then eventually you may be able to try a light diet and move on to a more normal diet.

However, for many, moving through these stages can be slow. Some people also require support feeding (see enteral feeding, pages 74 and 113), with a feeding tube into the gut or vein. Again, I trust this explains why being adequately nourished and built up before surgery is so important.

Nutritional issues involved in gastrointestinal cancers

As you might expect, there are often more challenges with a gastro-intestinal cancer, and individuals with this type of cancer benefit from being in close contact with the dietitian.

This type of cancer is often picked up because of unexplained weight loss, bleeding from the bowel, swallowing difficulties or a feeling of food getting caught in the gut. The most common mode of treatment is surgery, alongside chemotherapy or radiation either pre- or post-surgery or both. As you can imagine, once there is a tumour that needs to be removed from the mouth, throat, oesophagus, stomach, pancreas or small or large bowel, there are likely to be a number of nutritional challenges.

But before we consider them, here is some background on the usual role of the stomach.

I quite often refer to the stomach as being like a washing machine where various juices are released to moisten the semi-solid food mixtures, clean the food (by way of acids which help kill off bacteria) and regulate how quickly the contents move on to the next stage of digestion, which occurs in the small intestine. The stomach is also key to helping the body take up vitamin B12, iron and calcium. Essentially, it is a muscular bag that mixes food with acid. It also acts as a holding vat where there is almost a queuing system that allows certain food nutrients to move on to the next stage of digestion in an orderly and timely fashion, rather than just letting all the food rush through in a chaotic manner. The top part of the stomach is connected to the oesophagus and there is a regulating valve called a sphincter, which when working properly should stop the acid released in the stomach regurgi-tating into the oesophagus, causing acid reflux. The lower part of the stomach connects to the small bowel. This is where the food nutrients are moved to meet up with the digestive enzymes released from the pancreas. The enzymes allow food particles to be broken down into minute nutrients, so that they can move from the gut into the bloodstream and on to be used for energy and regeneration.

There are two types of approaches to stomach surgery: removing either only a part of the stomach (partial gastrectomy) or the whole lot (total gastrectomy). Other related surgeries are pancreatic surgery and oesophageal surgery, which basically involve a repiping of the gut, and this reworking can often affect function.

The main post-op problems are a smaller capacity in the stomach and the reduced ability to hold in the stomach contents at both ends. Think of the stomach as being like a mid-sized balloon which has had the air taken out of it. Imagine that there is a valve at the top (between the throat and the stomach) and another at the bottom (between the stomach and the small intestine); often the regulating ability of these valves is reduced.

Problems include feeling full (or early satiety) after eating or drinking; loss of appetite or reduced intake which causes weight loss; feelings of indigestion and or/reflux; and dumping syndrome, which is when the food contents rush through, causing a drop in blood sugar and urgent diarrhoea and vomiting.

Feeling full after eating and drinking

This is a problem everyone who has stomach surgery experiences. When we eat, the food goes into the stomach, and in preparation the stomach muscle wall relaxes to accommodate a meal as soon as you smell food or salivate at the sight of it. This is controlled by a nerve called the vagus nerve.

If an operation has made the stomach smaller or if it is scarred, it is less able to relax or stretch and the space available within it to hold a meal is greatly reduced. Sometimes, too, the vagus nerve is cut or damaged during surgery. Hence, after surgery, capacity is reduced and the ability of the stomach muscles to relax may also be reduced; this means that once you start eating and drinking and the food enters the stomach, it puts a lot more pressure on the stomach wall and causes it to distend. This makes you feel full, and at times uncomfortable, sooner than normal.

It is important to eat smaller, more regular meals and snacks. It is also better to eat less bulky meals, to reduce fibre intake and to boost the nutrient density and calorie content of foods to help you hold your weight. If you are having problems, discuss the details of your approach with your dietitian. It is also a good idea to ask about taking a multi-vitamin and mineral supplement as it can be very difficult to meet the recommended intakes. Additional supplements such as B12 and iron may also need to be prescribed (B12 needs to be injected directly into the bloodstream).

It is also best to drink around 30 minutes before or after meals, with small sips during the meal period. Too much fluid with meals only exacerbates the problem.

Reflux and indigestion

This is caused by the regurgitation or backward flow of the acidic stomach juices into the throat or oesophagus. Trapped wind can also be a cause of the burping or indigestion-type symptoms.

Ask your doctor for antacid medication, and again have small, lighter meals and regular snacks that incorporate some lean protein. Soft drinks, alcohol, spicy food, fatty foods and excessive amounts of fruit and vegetables all contribute to excess wind and indigestion.

Dumping syndrome

While not everyone experiences feelings of light-headedness, tummy cramps or diarrhoea after stomach surgery, these symptoms are often due to something called dumping syndrome. The symptoms can occur either within 30 minutes of eating a meal or several hours later. The initial type is called early dumping syndrome and happens when food rapidly enters the bowel. This draws fluid into the bowel from the surrounding organs and tissues and causes a drop in blood pressure.

Early dumping syndrome often gets better on its own over a few months. It can be reduced by eating slowly, choosing small, frequent, dry meals and having drinks between meals rather than during them.

It can also help not to overdo foods that are high in added sugars or higher GI foods. Or take foods with sugar mixed into a larger meal that includes some protein such as meat, chicken or fish, some grains like pasta, basmati rice and baby or new potatoes (lower GI) or some granary bread if you can tolerate it. It is also a good excuse to have a lie-down after a meal, as resting for 15–30 minutes immediately after eating can reduce the problem.

Dumping syndrome which usually occurs a couple of hours after meals or when a meal has been missed is referred to as late dumping syndrome. It is caused by the rapid movement of certain carbohydrates from the stomach through the small bowel and into the bloodstream. This causes a rapid rise in your blood sugar levels, which in turn causes the body to pump out large amounts of insulin, a hormone which is needed to take the glucose or sugar from your blood into your cells. However, what happens in this case is that the levels of insulin continue to increase even after the glucose or sugar levels begin to fall and you end up with low blood sugar, which causes the feelings of light-headedness, faintness and fatigue. The rush can also affect bowel function, contributing to cramps and diarrhoea.

Again, you will do better to eat smaller, more regular meals. These should include some higher biological value protein foods, and any higher sugar type foods should be taken with some slower-release or lower GI type carbohydrate foods such as durum wheat pasta, basmati rice, wholegrain pitta or bread, oats, etc. Eating food and drinking fluid at separate times can also help to prevent late dumping syndrome.

The main reason for giving you a little more detail on the nutritional management of stomach cancer is to encourage you to speak to your doctor or clinic if you are having problems with your diet or the symptoms that surround it. For some reason individuals are ready to report lots of other problems, but when it comes to the diet we are often quite stoical or think that we can sort it out ourselves.

With some professional dietetic guidance and support, most people find that, while dietary problems may not completely disappear, it is possible to learn to manage and work around them.

Some of the other problems around gut surgery which need to be monitored are:

- calcium malabsorption;
- anaemia caused by low iron, vitamin B12 deficiency;
- narrowing of the swallowing passages cause by scarring from surgery, which can make swallowing more difficult or cause foods like doughy bread to get caught;
- depression and mood swings (is there any wonder with all this going on!).

Diarrhoea

Diarrhoea is defined as an increase in the number and/or an increase in liquidity of the stools. There is not an exact number of stools per day that defines diarrhoea and it is something that is usually compared with the norm. It has many causes, including diet, stress, inflammation or irritation of the bowel wall or cell linings, certain treatments like radiation or chemotherapy to the abdomen or pelvis, and surgery in the stomach or bowel.

Diarrhoea is a common problem in cancer treatments that are targeted near or around the small or large bowel. It can also be a problem after any type of stomach or pancreatic surgery, especially if this has involved the vagus nerve. If the vagus nerve has been cut during surgery there is often a feeling of wanting to open your bowels quite urgently. This can cause considerable trauma, although the use of anti-diarrhoea medication such as Imodium can help. Your doctor or clinic can recommend what is best for you. You may need to take quite a hefty dose of Imodium tablets throughout the day if you are having regular bouts of diarrhoea.

Diarrhoea can happen in short episodes for a few days or weeks after surgery before the bowel returns to normal. Everyone is different, so it's difficult to predict how long it may last or how many times a day you'll get diarrhoea. Some people may have diarrhoea once a day, while others may have it a few times a day.

Food Fix – tips for coping with diarrhoea

- Avoid high-fibre food. Try low-fibre foods such as white bread and rice, pasta and potatoes without their skins.
- Drinking plenty of fluids to prevent dehydration is vital. If diarrhoea is severe, rehydration solution (see below) can be useful.
- Anti-diarrhoea medications prescribed by a doctor do help, and at times higher doses throughout the day are needed.
- Try to chew food well.
- Try to eat slowly.
- Try to relax or lie down after eating.
- Avoid spicy foods.
- Avoid fatty foods (except if the cause of the diarrhoea is dumping syndrome, which commonly occurs following gastric or oesophageal surgery).

- Avoid foods that are very hot or very cold.
- Limit tea, coffee or alcohol, especially if you find it aggravates the diarrhoea.
- A course of pre-biotics may help to restore levels of healthy bacteria in the gut which can be stripped out by diarrhoea. Pre-biotics like Bimuno® are safer during treatment as they provide the gut with food to feed the good bacteria currently present in the gut instead of introducing other types of foreign bacteria.
- Employing some of the dietary recommendations for irritable bowel syndrome (IBS) such as the low FODMAP diet can be explored. This has been shown to improve bowel function in individuals with IBS, and while more research is needed it can be worth discussing with your dietitian or a gastroenterologist whether a trial of such a diet would be helpful for the management of your type of diarrhoea. This really depends on whether diet is a factor or a cause in the diarrhoea.

In cases of severe diarrhoea due to bowel surgery, it is possible to become dehydrated very quickly as well as to lose mineral salts. It may be advisable to drink a rehydration solution such as Dioralyte, or you can make your own using the following recipe from St Mark's Hospital in London.

St Mark's oral rehydration solution

20 g (six level 5 ml spoons) glucose   3.5 g (one level 5 ml spoon)
2.5 g (one heaped 25 ml spoon)   sodium chloride (salt)
*   sodium bicarbonate*

Dissolve the ingredients in 1 litre of tap water and drink as required or prescribed. Two to three litres per day may be necessary to maintain hydration. A dash of sugar-free flavoured squash may be added to improve the flavour. Using a straw may also help.

If you are at risk of dehydration due to severe diarrhoea then you should use the oral rehydration solution instead of drinking regular fluids or water. It may be better to separate ingestion of fluids from the intake of foods.

The solution should be freshly prepared daily and stored in the refrigerator.

If you think you are becoming dehydrated you should contact your doctor or the specialist clinical team at your cancer centre.

Constipation

Constipation is a common side effect of chemotherapy and radio-therapy. The cause is often related to pain-control medications, along with the impact of certain treatment drugs. A starting point can be to experiment with building up your fibre intake. As outlined in the section on fibre (see page 52) it is important to balance fibre intake between soluble and insoluble types. I often say these fibres are like a marriage and the best results for the bowel come when they are consumed together: for example, wholegrain cereal + fruit, wholegrain pitta bread + salad, jacket potato + steamed vegetables.

There are times where the problems of constipation cannot be rectified by diet and you will need to use the laxative medications prescribed by your doctor or clinic. These medications should be used as instructed, as continuing constipation can result in feelings of discomfort and may even contribute to a loss of appetite or some nausea.

Food Fix – tips for coping with constipation

If your doctor has suggested you work on your diet to help manage your constipation, the following should be considered.

- Ensure you are eating enough wholegrain cereals such as Bran Flakes, All-Bran, and supermarket own-brand bran cereals. You may also need to increase your consumption of wholegrain bread, wholemeal pasta, brown rice and wholewheat crackers. Grain fibre is important to add bulk to stools, and this is what helps flush the system. However, if you have not been eating much fibre you should increase your intake gradually, and only if you can tolerate it.
- Try adding two teaspoons of flaxseeds daily to your diet, and gradually increase to one to two tablespoons. A good way to do this is to put the flaxseeds in yoghurt the night before to allow them to soften. Some people also enjoy them added to muesli,

and again you can prepare this the night before, adding milk so that it is easier to eat the next morning.

- Include at least five to seven servings of fruit and vegetables a day. Smoothies and soups can be a great way to do this.
- A soup with pulses like lentils or beans can be a delicious meal that is full of fibre. For example, lentil and tomato soup is a lovely spicy soup that's full of goodness yet is surprisingly light to eat. Serve it with a slice of sourdough, rye or granary bread to help inject more of the insoluble type of fibre.
- A sufficient fluid intake is vital; keep drinks to hand and sip throughout the day.
- Daily exercise can help: a walk in the park or whatever you are able to manage.
- If these suggestions aren't effective then discuss with your doctor a suitable bulking product or laxative.
- Individuals who have had a bowel obstruction or who are at risk should discuss the appropriate intake of fibre with their doctor or dietitian.
- If you have wind or bloating, limit foods such as broccoli, onion, garlic, cabbage, pulses, apples, carbonated drinks, sugar-free gum and sweets, and excessive amounts of refined wheat products. Any wind should improve if your bowels move properly.

Soft textures

Soft/purée diet

If you are having difficulty swallowing solid food you may need to follow a soft or purée textured diet. Foods should be solid but moist and easy to separate or mash with a fork. They should require little effort to chew and eat. If you require puréed foods, use a hand-held blender to ensure there are no lumps.

Preparing soft and puréed foods

- Add extra moisture to savoury dishes by adding a sauce, gravy or plain yoghurt.
- Add extra moisture to sweet dishes by adding a sauce, custard, yoghurt, cream or milk.
- Foods should be soft enough to mash with a fork or masher.

Foods to avoid

- Stringy, fibrous textures, e.g. celery, lettuce and runner beans.
- Skins and husks, e.g. those on beans, peas, grapes and sweet corn, poultry.
- Crumbly, dry foods, e.g. toast, bread crusts, flaky pastry, dry biscuits and crisps.
- Hard foods, e.g. nuts, seeds, dried fruit, tough meats and gristle.
- Bread can also be difficult to swallow.

Finding a balance

- It is important that your soft diet contains all the nutrients you need in order to prevent weight loss, as many people who have difficulties swallowing are only able to eat a small amount at one time.
- Eating six small meals or three meals and three snacks (or supplement drinks) each day can help.
- Weigh yourself once a week on the same set of scales and keep a record of your weight. If you have lost weight or are finding

Table 7.1 Tips for soft foods

Food group	Tips for soft diet and fortifying foods
Protein foods Meat, poultry, fish, soya mince, tofu, Quorn, eggs and pulses	Minced meat, soya mince, corned beef hash, skinless sausages, bolognese sauce, cottage pie, shepherd's pie, fish pie, kedgeree, hotpots and casseroles are all suitable (purée if necessary). Serve with gravy or a savoury sauce such as white, cheese, parsley or tomato (use fortified milk to make the sauces). Fish may contain bones – take care, and flake before serving with a sauce, or use tinned fish. Poached, fried and boiled eggs are suitable if the yolk and white are solid. Add cheese to scrambled egg and omelette. Beans, pulses and lentils should be cooked until soft, or use tinned varieties. Serve with a soup or sauce, e.g. dhal.

Food group	Tips for soft diet and fortifying foods
Milk and dairy (for calcium and protein) Whole milk, yoghurt, fromage frais, cheese and cream	Fortify full-cream milk, by adding 4 tablespoons of skimmed milk powder to 1 pint of milk. Keep in the fridge and use this to make soups, sauces and puddings, milkshakes, fruit smoothies or hot milk drinks for between meals. Add full-fat cheese and yoghurt to sauces, soups, potatoes and vegetables. Cream, Evaporated Milk, custard and ice cream are useful to add to puddings and fruit to add moisture. Add jam or honey for extra energy. Home-made, tinned or instant puddings such as sponge, semolina, ice cream, mousse, milk jelly, rice, tapioca, crème caramel, yoghurt and fromage frais are suitable.
Carbohydrates (for energy and vitamins) Breads, cereals and potatoes	Avoid warm fresh bread as it forms lumps. Cook pasta until soft and serve with a sauce; try with bolognaise, cream or cheese sauces. Tinned pasta is also soft. Cook potatoes until soft then mash using fortified milk and butter (or margarine) or try instant mash with fortified milk. Serve jacket potatoes with a soft filling, e.g. baked beans (purée if needed). Make instant oat cereal or Weetabix with fortified milk for breakfast or a quick snack.
Fruit and vegetables (for vitamins, minerals and fibre) Juice: fresh, tinned or frozen varieties	Cook vegetables until soft. Chop, mash or purée. Add stock, sauce, fortified milk, margarine, olive oil, cheese, cream or sour cream to vegetables for moisture. Do not use stringy vegetables or those with pips, skins or seeds. Tinned and stewed fruits are suitable. Fresh fruit should be peeled and seeds removed (e.g. use soft fruit such as banana or mango). Drink a glass of fruit or vegetable juice daily for vitamin C.

it difficult to eat enough you may benefit from fortifying your foods. Ask your dietitian or doctor if this will be of benefit to you.

- Drinking six to eight glasses of fluid daily is important to help alleviate or prevent constipation. Having one glass of fruit or vegetable juice helps, as do tinned or soft fruit (e.g. prunes) and wholegrain cereals such as porridge or smoothies that include a cereal such as All-Bran (blended).

Include foods from each of the food groups at each mealtime and fortify foods to ensure you have a balanced diet with all the nutrients you need. Table 7.1 will give you more ideas.

Meal ideas

Breakfast

- Porridge or instant hot oat cereal
- Cereals soaked in hot or cold milk, e.g. Weetabix
- Scrambled eggs with extra milk and margarine.

Main meal

- Dishes made with minced meat, e.g. shepherd's pie
- Pies with soft filling, e.g. cheese and potato pie
- Stews, casseroles and mornays
- Poached or grilled fish, e.g. plaice, haddock, salmon, tuna
- Egg-based dishes, e.g. scrambled eggs, omelettes
- Pasta with sauces, e.g. macaroni cheese, spaghetti bolognese, ravioli
- Soft ready-meals
- Dhal and hummus
- Pancakes with soft fillings, e.g. mince, fish, melted cheese and sauces
- Savoury mousse.

Vegetables

All vegetables should be well cooked or mashed.

- Boiled carrots and swede
- Boiled/mashed potatoes
- Boiled broccoli heads and cauliflower florets
- Cauliflower cheese.

Sweet dishes

- Puréed or stewed fruit, e.g. apples, pears, prunes, banana and mango served with custard, cream or ice cream
- Fruit fools
- Yoghurt – especially thick creamy varieties, e.g. Greek yoghurt
- Milk-based puddings, e.g. rice pudding, egg custard, crème caramel
- Mousses, jellies and ice cream.

Nourishing drinks

- Nutritional supplement drinks provide a concentrated amount of energy, protein, vitamins and minerals in a small volume. Many varieties of milk and juice type supplements are available on prescription.

Fortified powdered drinks and soups can be bought from the chemist, e.g. Complan or Build-up. See the section on nourishing drinks (page 104) for more information on these types of products.

The brew

The brew is a recipe shared by Dr Greg Cox, who is a dietitian working with endurance and Olympic athletes at the Australian Institute of Sport. This is a great way to boost the humble but very versatile potato.

1 or 2 large potatoes (you can also mix in sweet potatoes)
1 generous tablespoon butter
¼–½ cup full-cream, high protein milk
Pinch salt

1 tablespoon Polycose, Polyjoule or Maxijul powder or Pro-Cal shot or other high protein supplement
1 teaspoon Bovril, or to taste, or ¼ chicken stock cube

Prepare some mashed potato using the potatoes, butter and high protein milk (or make a batch of instant mashed potato). Mix in 2 tablespoons of your preferred energy supplement and additional flavours such as chicken stock or some Bovril.

Loss of appetite and building up

Struggling with a poor appetite is a difficult side effect for many individuals in treatment for cancer. As previously outlined, there are many reasons why your appetite may be affected, including the cancer-induced wasting state, cachexia. While it can be extremely difficult to eat to meet your energy requirements, if you want to build up you do need to eat more than your body is using. For many, this means aiming at 2,500–3,000 kcal a day. Typically individuals with little or no appetite will be lucky if they are taking in 800–1,400 kcal a day. It is no wonder the weight drops away.

If you have little or no interest in eating it is important to organize a strict diet routine. It is usually better to nibble or pick your way through lots of regular (one to two hourly) mini-meals or snacks. One of our consultants tells his patients to try and put something into their mouths every hour or to keep a handful of sweets or chocolates in their pockets. Do experiment with lots of extra special small meals and snack treats. It can also be easier to drink a high-calorie formula drink (see page 103).

Food Fix – tips for building up and coping when you do not feel like eating much

- Try to eat or at least nibble 'little and often', having more snacks. Instead of three meals a day, try to eat every two to three hours or have six snack type meals a day.
- Try to eat more nourishing snacks like eggs, cheese, fish like smoked salmon, minced meat pasta meals, nuts, peanut butter on toast, wholegrain crackers or a bowl of cereal with milk, milk-shakes, scones or a piece of appetizing cake. Use high protein milk rather than regular milk.
- Eat puddings and desserts after a break following the main course. Rice puddings with a little extra cream can work well.
- If the smell of food affects your appetite, try to have foods that are slightly warm or cold, such as quiche, smoked salmon, cheese, rice pudding, etc.
- Have small servings of favourite foods in stock. It is a good time to indulge in something a little special that may help tempt your taste buds: a sharp cheddar, a silky mousse or some delicious smoked salmon on a slice of rye with some mascarpone.

- Serve food in small portions – seeing and being expected to eat large portions may further reduce appetite. The reheat meals designed for young children, like shepherd's pie, bolognese and macaroni cheese, are worth trying.
- Ensure a stock of easy-to-make foods are in the cupboard, like soup, and reheat or tasty frozen meals either bought in or home-made from any leftovers. This is something to ask family and friends to help with.
- Try to avoid drinking water or too much liquid before and during a meal, as this may fill the stomach with liquids instead of more nutritious foods.
- Sip nutritious drinks throughout the day, like milky or sugary drinks.
- Try a small glass of good wine, sherry or spirits just before eating, as this can help to stimulate appetite.
- Try a short walk in the fresh air before eating or open a window for some fresh air if the weather is not too cold.
- Make the table or tray look attractive with a tablecloth or some flowers.
- Keep nutritious little snacks to hand throughout the day like nuts, cereal bars, yoghurts, cheese sticks, dried fruit, etc.
- Make the most of times when appetite is at its best, often in the mornings. Perhaps try scrambled or poached egg on toast with some bacon.
- Try eating a meal or snack in front of the television or with the radio on in the background – people naturally tend to eat more when there is some form of distraction around them. It's rather like the 1,000 kcal box of popcorn that many get through at a movie.
- Use some of the high-calorie supplement drinks. You can make these yourself using high protein milk, or talk to your clinic and the dietitian about trying out the supplements available on the NHS. I know that at first many people like the idea of replacing meals with a supplement drink; however, these drinks are quite rich in taste and many people find them sweet. The trick to taking these drinks is to chill them and then decant them into a nice glass instead of the box or bottle they come in. I also rec-ommend some ice and a straw, as it can be easier to sip slowly on them.

Nutrition sip drinks or food supplements

How to use these products

One way to boost your nutrition and help you keep the weight on is to take some extra high-calorie drinks or to use energy, protein and/or nutrition type powder bases to bump up the nutrition and energy concentration of the food you are able to manage.

Now, for some odd reason I used to imagine how I might advertise these products if given charge of the marketing budget for one of the companies producing these supplement drinks. One of the ideas I came up with was a big picture of plate of food with some meat, vegetables, potato, a glass of milk and a piece of bread all being captured and flowing into the supplement bottle. Another thought was to insert a number of different straws, labelled with vitamins, minerals, carbohydrates, proteins and fats. Essentially I was trying to portray that some of the nutrition supplement drinks can work as mini-meal substitutes or as a nourishing between-meal top-up. The value in using these products is that they can be a convenient power-pack injection of nutrition.

In addition to experimenting with your own formulations, there are more and more commercial products appearing on the market. In fact, the current range now resembles the breakfast cereal aisle in the supermarket. In addition to several brand options, there is a wide range of presentations, flavours, concentrations and consistencies. Some are milk-like, juice-like or yoghurt-like in flavour. Some have a thicker consistency, to help with swallowing. Some are fruit-based or pudding-like. There is a wide range of nutritional formulations. On the top shelf are the products which are referred to as 'complete feeds'. This means that if you consumed enough to provide for your fluid and energy requirements, you could live on them. They are basically formulated to provide for all the nutritional needs of the body. The next tier are a group which provide what is described as a 'complete source of nutrition'. This means they provide almost all of the nutrients your body needs and are ideal as top-up or build-up drinks to be taken around mealtimes. Some of these products have fibre added to help the bowels work properly, while there is a new range which is formulated like rocket fuel, providing a super-concentrated source of energy and/or protein. These come in a shot presentation or in small-volume bottles. Other products provide only carbohydrate or fat or protein supplements.

The energy density or amount of calories provided per ml is also something which ranges between different products and brands. Generally they start at around 1 kcal/g and build up to the very concentrated types which can provide around 3–4 kcal/ml. To put this in context, something like Coca-Cola provides around 0.4 kcal/ml, so on a ml to ml basis these drinks give you a lot more bang for your buck.

There is also an emerging specialist product range. Some of these products are designed to be consumed to build up for surgery, some are for specific digestive issues and others are for certain advanced types of cancer.

Some people like to experiment with the supplements on the market for sports people, those from health food stores or those designed to help people 'bulk muscle up'. In most cases there is no problem with trying out some of these products, although it is essential that you check with the clinic team, dietitian, pharmacist or doctor to ensure there are no contra-indications. I often use some of these products with some of my younger or usually active clients; they often prefer to use the products they can get from a bike shop or gym and then to focus on more of a build-up or fitness type goal instead of one just centred around their treatment.

Points to consider before you start these products

Whatever the nutritional issue or the reason for thinking about employing nutritional supplement drinks, there are certain points you should consider first. The most important starting point will be to look at the baseline diet to estimate what your current nutritional intake is and whether your diet is best supporting you, as well as maximizing your food or calorie intake.

1 Are you able to eat, chew and safely swallow and digest normal food?
2 If so, what type of foods are you eating, and are your dietary patterns best for supporting you and any issues you may be struggling with? For example, are you still trying to eat a healthy, low-fat, low-sugar diet that incorporates lots of fruits

and vegetables, when in fact you may be needing to focus on more of the higher-calorie or higher-protein foods?

3 Are you taking small meals with extra nourishing snacks? For example, are you trying to put a small snack or nibble into your mouth every hour or two?

4 Are there any treats or different types of foods that might tempt you? For example, do you enjoy olives from a deli, a special piece of cheese with a cracker, smoked Scottish salmon with some lemon and mascarpone, a scone with jam and cream, a piece of crumbly carrot cake . . .?

5 Are there any ways you could add extra calories to the food you like? Have you tried high protein milk, some extra butter on your food, mixing some peanut butter into a stir-fry . . .?

6 Have you had a look at some of the Food Fix suggestions to help deal with any treatment side effects or issues? (See pages 76, 81, 85, 94, 96 and 102.)

7 How do you get on making your own nutrition supplement drinks? Is this something you would like or can manage?

Once these questions have been considered, tried, tested or discussed with your clinic team and/or the dietitian, it is also a good idea to look at whether a trial of some nutrition supplement drinks or powders would give you that extra edge, or at least help you out.

These products can be expensive and so I recommend you either discuss a supply on prescription or organize some trial or sample products. This can be worth doing before you go out and buy a month's supply. Wastage is a big issue with these products, and more often than not the reason is that they don't agree with or suit the user. I know many people who have ended up with a cupboard full of products which they bought only to find them not to their taste. Often, nutrition supplement drinks are handed out like a miracle solution. However, when your appetite is compromised they can be just as difficult, if not harder, to take than your regular meals.

It needs to be understood that they must be used in the context of your drugs, treatments and general diet. All too often I see people who have been handed a box of supplement drinks that are not to their taste or whose baseline diet is not doing anything to help them. When they see me it turns out that no one has really explained how they could modify their diet, worked out the nutritional shortfalls or discussed the use of these products within the context of their treatment and nutritional goals.

It is important to think about and/or write down your treatment and nutritional goals. Dietitians keep up to date with the range of products available, including any new ones. So your dietitian is the best person to ask for further advice if you have been recommended a product that has not been to your taste. If you have any other health issues, such as diabetes or kidney or liver trouble, then it is essential that you consult a dietitian or doctor as the extra carbohydrate or protein in such drinks needs to be factored in to the overall management of these conditions.

You also need to be clear in your mind about the use of these products, and to remember what they are for. Yes, at times they can be difficult to drink and difficult to get down, but keep in mind that their sole purpose is to give you the fuel and extra nutrients you need to motor on through the treatments. So although they can be difficult to slog through, the benefits as regards your energy and nutritional health will help to make the effort worthwhile.

Bear in mind also that most of the companies who produce these supplements have websites which provide recipe ideas. Sometimes it can be easier to take the products as a cake, biscuit, pudding or home-made smoothie.

The range

It all depends on your need, tastes and ability to cook, shop and prepare your own supplement drinks. I work around the following options for nutrition supplements if it is felt such products might be helpful:

- You could make your own.
- Nutritionally fortified drinks, soups or desserts can be used as in-between drinks or taken with meals. These may be:
  - nutritionally balanced – high protein, high energy, nutritionally fortified (to be used as a top-up drink, in conjunction with other foods);
  - complete varieties – high energy, high protein, nutritionally fortified to be a complete source of nutrition (you can live on these drinks);

- energy concentrated drinks – smaller volume, concentrated food supplements with very high energy concentrations, suitable for individuals who prefer smaller, concentrated volumes;
- supplement drinks indicated for specialist feed indications such as lung and pancreatic cancer or for digestive difficulties. These products are very specialized and would be recommended by your doctor or dietitian.

• Energy or protein powders or formulas can be added to water or milk or soft or liquid foods. These products are designed as a convenient option for adding extra calories and protein to your food.

• Some sports nutrition formulas and drinks are available in bike shops, health food stores and gyms. These products are readily available and can be used to add extra energy and protein to your food. While they are suitable, you should be aware they can be more expensive and are not available on prescription.

Making your own

It is really easy to put together a range of energy-boosting supplement drinks. All you need is something to liquidize the mixture, such as a hand-held or jug blender.

Basic ingredients can include milk (including high protein milk drink), fruit juice, fruits such as banana or berries (frozen varieties are great), yoghurt, ice cream, chocolate or strawberry sauce, crushed ice. For fibre top-ups, add a tablespoon or two of a bran type cereal such as All-Bran, a Weetabix or 1–2 tablespoons of flaxseeds. This can be helpful if you are reliant on a soft or liquid diet. It is also possible to use the commercial powder type supplements as a base for making up a drink that is better suited to your palate.

Some ideas

• Fruit salad smoothie: 1 cup high protein milk, 1 cup of mixed fruit salad (¼ cup grapes, ¼ cup melon, ¼ cup pineapple, ¼ cup apple), ¼ cup pineapple or orange juice, 1 scoop ice cream (try a mix of frozen fruits or a pot of fruit salad from the supermarket).

• Berry smoothie: ½ cup milk or water (use high protein milk), ¼ cup yoghurt or ice cream, 1 cup mixed frozen berries (or fresh if you have them).

- Almond or cashew milk: 3 cups water, 1 cup raw almonds or cashews, sugar to taste (optional). Using a powerful blender, mix on high for 2 minutes. You may need to strain the sediment or push the milk through a sieve, though this is not needed if you are using cashews. This milk can be used as an alternative to regular milk; however, be aware that the calcium level is low and so unless you are taking a supplement it should not be used as a permanent replacement drink.
- Another refreshing, nut-flavoured smoothie drink is made with peanut butter. Add 1 banana broken into chunks, 1 cup milk, ¼ cup peanut butter, 1 tablespoon honey and 1 cup ice cubes. Place bananas, milk, peanut butter, honey and ice cubes in a blender; blend until smooth, about 30 seconds.
- Super-green smoothie: ¼ cup water or milk, ¼ cup pineapple juice, 1 cup green grapes, ¼ of a ripe pear, ¼ of an avocado (peeled with stone removed), 1 cup broccoli florets, ¼ cup washed spinach, ½ cup ice cubes. Place all ingredients in a blender and mix for 1 minute.
- For a savoury or tart taste bud kick, try a plain yoghurt lassi. Mix ½ cup water, ½ cup plain yoghurt, ¼–½ teaspoon salt, 2 teaspoons sugar, ¼ cup ice cubes.
- When the taste buds are getting a little tired of sweet tastes, try a good old-fashioned iced coffee. Put ½–1 teaspoon of instant coffee granules into a tall glass, dissolve the coffee in 1–2 table-spoons of boiling water, mix in a scoop of ice cream and fill the glass with some cold milk.
- Soup bases such as Heinz tomato soup, which is a taste that often appeals to challenged taste buds, mix well with some high protein milk and a scoop of a neutral or vanilla-based supplement powders such as Complan or Build-up.
- See the Brew recipe (page 101) for preparing a super-boost mashed potato.

You can add one to two tablespoons of a nutrition supplement powder such as Enshake or Calshake to all these drinks.

Ready-to-drink products, soups or desserts (liquid supplements)

'Nutritionally complete' drink or meal supplements

These products contain the nutrients to replace a meal. Your doctor or dietitian can prescribe them, or ask your clinic or district nurse. It's also possible to buy them yourself without a prescription and there are a number of companies selling them through the internet. Even if you use these products independently, you should still be monitored by your doctor or dietitian, especially if you are having difficulties.

There are many presentations of these products, including liquid in a carton or bottle, and they may be either milkshake style or fruit juice style. There are products with added fibre and highly concentrated, smaller-bottle presentations as well.

Please refer to Table A.1 in the Appendix (see page 146) for a snapshot of the product ranges, flavours, energy and protein levels available.

The core or starter range products are:

- milk-based
  - Ensure Plus
  - Fresubin Energy
  - Fortisip
  - Resource Shake
- fruit-based
  - Ensure Plus Juice
  - Fortijuice
  - Fresubin Jucy
  - Resource Fruit.

Each of the brands above also has a fibre-enriched version in its range. The fibre-enriched products may be preferable if you are not managing to consume enough fibre and/or are experiencing problems with your bowels. This should be discussed with your clinic team.

Also included in these product ranges are higher-calorie or more concentrated, smaller-volume presentations, soups, desserts and yoghurt-flavoured drinks. Each brand offers a wide range of flavour options.

In most cases you have these between meals and carry on with your normal diet as well. Drinking between two and three cartons a day gives a substantial boost to your overall nutritional intake as they provide around 300 kcal per carton. Alternatively they can be used as meal replacements: in general, two cartons would provide around 600 kcal, and if you can take three over the day they would provide 900 kcal. Again, you need to discuss with the doctor or dietitian the quantity required to meet your individual nutritional needs at this time.

Balanced supplement drinks with added vitamins and minerals

These are a useful range of supplements, which are readily available over the counter from most larger pharmacies and in some of the bigger supermarkets. They come as a box of individual powder sachets. There are options to make them up as milkshakes, soups, hot drinks or cold drinks. They provide an ideal nutritional top-up either between meals or alongside your main meal, especially if you find a soup or a milkshake easier to take than a full plate of food.

They include products such as:

- Build-up – soups and milkshakes
- Complan – soups and milkshakes.

Very high energy, nutritionally balanced powders that can be mixed with milk or water

These products are essentially a heavy-duty version of the balanced supplement drinks above. When mixed with milk they can provide up to 600 kcal per serving. They are available on prescription or can be ordered by your pharmacist.

- Scandishake – box of sachets
- Enshake – box of sachets
- Calshake – box of sachets.

Energy or protein powder or liquids

Using some of these products gives you lots of opportunities to be creative and boost the energy and protein you get from each bite or sip you take. There are many companies who now provide a range of reasonably taste-free high protein and energy powders and liquids. Use some of the recipes included in this chapter or add them to your own family favourites.

The range of products is outlined below.

- Energy powders – neutral-flavoured carbohydrate supplements that can be used to top up calories in most foods and beverages, and can even be added to a humble cup of tea:
  - Polycal – 400 g tin
  - Maxijul – 200 g tin
  - Polycose – 350 g tin
  - Vitajoule – 200 g tin
  - Caloreen – 500 g tin.
- Protein powders and gels:
  - Maxpro – 225 g tin
  - Protifar – 225 g tin
  - Vitapro – 250 g tin.
- Energy and protein gels or liquids:
  - Prosource – 30 ml gel-like sachets
  - Pro-Cal shots – 30 or 60 ml shot doses.

Protein-only powders are useful if you are eating reasonably well but need a boost in protein intakes; however, to gain the benefit of the added protein you also need to meet your energy requirements or else the protein will be used as a calorie or energy source. There are also potential problems from ingesting too much protein, especially if you have any kidney or liver problems. When using such products it is best to talk to the dietitian or your doctor about what amounts you should be taking.

When eating is just not enough

At times, owing to the location of the tumour, the impact of surgery and/or the intensity or side effects of treatment, eating is just not possible or is not going to be enough on its own to support your nutritional needs. This is when alternative support feeding needs to be considered. While this may well feel daunting, be reassured that support feeding is a regular, sometimes essential part of the treatment process. Quite often people who are initially upset at the idea of support feeding go on to be some of its biggest advocates. It can actually be a big relief to have this type of feeding as a back-up when eating and drinking is not easy or enjoyable and you have been unable to maintain your energy levels or weight despite your very best efforts. It is also the best option in many types of head and neck cancer, when it is difficult to eat properly or swallow as you normally would.

The first and preferable option for support feeding is enteral feeding. There are many ways to implement this, and all involve placement of a small tube in the gut to enable various formula feeds to be dripped in slowly or to be given in a bolus-type fashion. The simplest is to insert a thin feeding tube through the nose and into the stomach (nasogastric feeding). Another variation is to use a longer tube and to insert it a little further down the gut into the small intestine. The options here are nasoduodenal or nasojejunal. This way of feeding would be explored if there were extreme nausea or vomiting or digestion of the feeds further up the bowel. The other option, which is much more comfortable and discreet, is either percutaneous endoscopic gastrostomy feeding (known as a PEG) or radiologically inserted gastrostomy feeding (a RIG). This requires a small tube to be placed directly into the stomach wall, with variations that allow the feeding tube to be inserted further down the bowel into the duodenum or jejunum. The PEG or the RIG is usually employed if support feeding is required for longer than a few weeks.

The enteral method should always be employed as the first choice for support feeding, as physiologically it is the normal way to feed, and the bowel responds and works better in its immune support role when it is receiving a direct source of nutrition moving through it. The bowel is rather like a muscle: if it is rested for long periods its function and ability to defend the body from outside organisms will be compromised.

However, there are occasions when the bowel is not working properly and does need some time out. The type of feeding which is then employed is called parenteral nutrition. Parenteral feeding is when nutrition is fed through a drip directly into the bloodstream (via an intravenous tube called a central line, which may start in the arm but is generally moved to a larger vein in the chest). This method of feeding is quite complex and normally overseen by a team including the dietitian, pharmacist, nurse and doctor, who closely monitor your blood results to see how you are tolerating the feed and whether electrolytes or nutrients need to be added or reduced.

Support feeding at home

Once you are doing well and tolerating your feed regime, both enteral and parenteral feed regimes can be prepared for home use. However, before this you would be given lots of support, training and guidance on how to use the equipment and administer the formulas. The formula companies have a home nutrition support team who visit at home, and across each borough community nurses and dietitians can provide continuing guidance and support. Most hospital dietitians also provide contact numbers and emails. Again, this may seem daunting for you and your loved ones; however, many people, including children, go on to live quite normal lives feeding at home in this way. Again, the gains of better nutritional health, even if it has to be obtained in a different way, far exceed the potential complications of poor nutritional health and the stress around eating when you are in pain, just can't manage or are facing safety risks.

Stocking the pantry

Quite often I have found it easier (or have wanted) to just take people down to the supermarket to show them how to fill their trolley with more of the foods they need to eat at this time. In fact, over the years I have done this quite often with individuals I have worked with, and I find it is one of the most useful sessions we have together. I like to be practical, and you cannot get more practical than pushing the trolley around the aisle pointing out which foods to choose. I also like to help people look at food labels and to hone their food detective skills. This also gives them the confidence to know that their choices are supporting them better in their treatment and nutrition goals.

As a trained and keen cook, I also pride myself on my ability to suggest new food ideas and inspire people who are struggling with appetite, taste issues or other problems. This often means having to push them towards what might be unfamiliar food territory, and I understand how hard it can be for people to feel comfortable when they are not used to eating in a certain way.

To help you, Table 7.2 suggests what you might choose to put into a trolley that is trying to build you up and boost you, or one that is trying to keep you strong and well while also protecting you and helping you maintain a healthy weight.

Table 7.2 Build-up trolley v. weight-management trolley

Category	Build-up territory (stay strong and build up or help prevent further weight loss)	Healthy-treatment eating (stay strong but maintain your weight)
Fruit	Bananas, frozen or fresh berries (ideal for smoothies), pineapple (good for strange tastes in the mouth), tinned fruits, apples or pears or rhubarb for stewing, fruit juice, tomato juice, grapes, dried fruit e.g. apricots, tomatoes (pasta sauces, fresh and tinned).	Red berries (fresh or frozen), melons, citrus fruits like oranges, mandarins and clementines (except grapefruit if it has to be avoided), dark stone fruit like plums and cherries, nectarines, peaches, tomatoes, pomegranates, pineapple, apples, pears, papaya, etc.
Vegetables	Potatoes (including sweet), pumpkin, swede, turnip (all good for soft roasted veg or soups or mashed), frozen vegetable mixes, dark leafy green vegetables such as spinach, cucumber, mushrooms (great on toast), beetroot (great roasted or in soups), vegetable soups, carrots.	Dark leafy vegetables, broccoli, cauliflower, cabbage (try different colours), asparagus, peppers, fennel, garlic, onion, vegetable soups with pulses if you can tolerate them, carrots.
Dairy	Full-fat milk, yoghurts, dairy desserts such as chocolate mousse, rice pudding, cream, ice cream, sweetened condensed milk, cheese (try some treat options).	Low-fat dairy foods, cottage cheese (high in whey protein), yoghurt (check if probiotic is suitable), slivers of good-quality cheese.
Protein foods	Quality cuts, well-sourced red meat, offal e.g. kidneys, poultry, fish, pork, eggs, pre-prepared meals in supermarket (fresh or frozen) such as shepherd's pie, pasties, macaroni cheese, spaghetti bolognese, lasagne, Chinese dishes, stews or Indian curry, etc.	Lean red meat (treatment phase), poultry, fish, pork, eggs, additional whey protein supplements (may be the preferred option if muscle build-up a goal), healthier calorie-controlled pre-prepared meals, pulses such as Puy lentils, other canned and dried pulses.

(continued)

Table 7.2 *continued*

Category	Build-up territory (stay strong and build up or help prevent further weight loss)	Healthy-treatment eating (stay strong but maintain your weight)
Fats and oils	Nuts, nut butters (peanut, cashew, almond, etc.), extra-virgin olive oil for dressing food, rapeseed or vegetable oil for cooking, hemp oil, walnut or sesame oils, butter or margarine.	Limit intakes and choose small amounts of quality olive oils, vegetable or other nut oils. Choose an olive oil- or canola-based margarine or small scrapes of butter.
Cereal and grain foods	Bakery loaves, pitta, wraps, pasta, rice, risotto rice, pre-prepared dry and fresh rice and pasta mixes, pot noodles, potatoes, scones, pikelets, English muffins, crackers or biscuits (easier to swallow). Healthy protein-based take-out sandwiches, e.g. egg, cheese, chicken or lean meat.	Wholegrain or granary breads or pitta. Wholemeal wraps, dark cracker breads, sourdough or rye or spelt breads, quinoa, brown rice or pastas, risotto rice. White equivalents are suitable if easier to tolerate; however the satiety levels from these products will be lower.
Flavours and condiments	Soy sauce, fish sauce, oyster sauce, ketchup, jars of green and black olives, vinegars, horseradish cream, Dijon or wholegrain mustard and (if you can manage it) English mustard.	
Herbs and spices	Both trolleys should contain lots of fresh and/or dried herbs, spices and other natural flavours such as lemon, lime and pepper to enhance the food for both the taste and health boost needs. Refer to the herbs suggestions (see Table 5.4, pages 69–70) which encourage the use of mint, coriander, basil, rosemary, chives, parsley, thyme, turmeric, curcumin, lemon grass and garlic as everyday additions. A herb garden or a window box or terracotta pot is a great investment.	
Alcohol	A small glass of something can be used to help stimulate appetite and improve mealtime experience if alcohol is something you can tolerate or have the taste for. Many prefer sweeter wines or spirits. Why not open that special bottle with a friend or loved one? You can put the cork on an unfinished bottle and store in the fridge for another time.	Alcohol is a concentrated source of calories and is associated with many cancers. If you have a history of high alcohol intake then this is a good time to moderate and focus on quality, not quantity. Follow the WCRF guideline (page 16) if you do drink, then limit this to two drinks a day for men and one a day for women.

Category	Build-up territory (stay strong and build up or help prevent further weight loss)	Healthy-treatment eating (stay strong but maintain your weight)
Extra treats	Olives, dips, nuts, fun-sized chocolate, dark chocolate, take-out milk or thick shakes, sundaes, ice cream, cakes, biscuits (I prefer better quality or home-made if available, where you can added extra protein powders or skim milk), hot chocolate with the trimmings, home-made and bought puddings such as cheesecake, meringues.	Home-made popcorn cooked in the microwave, oat cakes, good quality fruit, malt loaf, bran muffins, low-fat Greek yoghurts, small square of dark chocolate, low-fat hot chocolate, small handful of nuts, protein-enriched milk drink (low-fat milk) or smoothie.
Equipment	Freezer, fridge, hand-held blender, good frying pan, small storage containers for freezing, slow cooker, microwave.	

8

Food safety and preventing infections

Food hygiene

Food safety, always important, is even more so for people during or after cancer treatment. Chemotherapy and radiotherapy take their toll on the immune system, so your body has to work harder to fight infection. In particular, you may be more vulnerable to food poisoning, and less able to cope with symptoms such as diarrhoea and vomiting.

Hygiene tips

- Wash your hands thoroughly before handling food, particularly between the fingers and under nails. A good tip is to keep washing until you have sung 'Happy Birthday' through twice (under your breath if you prefer). See the box on page 119 for more detailed instructions. There is also a seven-step hand-washing guide available on the internet (see http://www.uhb.nhs.uk/Downloads/pi/PiHandWashing.htm#Se).
- Keep pets out of the kitchen.
- Clean chopping boards and cooking utensils thoroughly, and use different boards for raw meat and vegetables.
- Consider investing in a dishwasher if you don't have one to ensure that eating and cooking utensils are thoroughly cleaned. If you wash up by hand, this means rinsing items under very hot water before leaving to dry.
- Clean work surfaces scrupulously with antibacterial detergent or a water and bleach solution, and replace sponges and cloths regularly.
- Wash all fruit and vegetables, even those labelled organic.
- Rinse cans before opening them.
- Think about investing in a water filter if you haven't already got one. This can reduce the amount of metals you consume in the

water. Filtered water also has a higher pH, which is better for your body.

Handwashing

Proper handwashing requires soap and water. Rubbing with soap breaks down the grease and dirt that carry most germs. Washing your hands for at least 15 to 30 seconds with soap and water not only makes your hands smell fresh but also reduces germ counts by up to 99 per cent.

Follow these eight simple steps to keep your hands clean:

1 palm to palm
2 between fingers
3 back of hands
4 base of thumbs
5 back of fingers
6 fingernails
7 wrists
8 rinse and wipe dry.

If you're at the clinic or hospital, or at the shops, it is important to use hand disinfectants as an extra hygiene measure after washing your hands with soap. The most common form of disinfectants are alcohol-based ones.

Ideally, wash your hands to make sure all dirt is removed as alcohol-based disinfectants work best on clean skin.

- Dry your hands.
- Apply an amount of disinfectant about the size of a coin to your hands. Rub them together, ensuring that both hands are covered with disinfectant, including the area under your nails.
- Keep rubbing for about 15 seconds, or until your hands feel dry.

Handling food

- Cook meat and eggs thoroughly.
- If you are storing food, let it cool and put it into the fridge. Ensure that anything reheated is piping hot inside before it is eaten. It should be warmer than 70° C.
- Keep raw meat, poultry and fish away from other food, and if possible keep a separate cutting board for these foods. Raw food should also be stored below cooked food in the fridge to minimize risk of drip contamination.
- Rotate food in the fridge and be extra careful about getting rid of food that may be past its best. Have a three or four day rule for

leftovers – throw out anything not eaten by then. Do also regularly check 'use by' or 'best before' dates on packages and tins.

Foods to avoid

If your immune system is low, you may need to take extra care about eating certain foods. Again, if you're not sure, do discuss this with your doctor or dietitian, and don't restrict whole food groups unnecessarily.

Some foods, however, carry a greater risk of food poisoning. They may more easily become prey to bacteria such as listeria, *E. coli* and salmonella. So do avoid:

- raw fish or shellfish, such as sushi and uncooked oysters;
- unpasteurized or raw milk, cheeses, yoghurts and other unpasteurized milk products. Cheeses are usually soft and include blue cheese, Brie, Camembert, feta, goat's cheese and ricotta;
- uncooked liver pâté;
- dry-cured, uncooked salami;
- cold smoked raw fish;
- cold hot dogs (heat thoroughly if you are going to eat);
- ready-prepared salads at supermarkets or delicatessens, especially if they contain egg, ham, chicken or seafood;
- raw or undercooked beef and other meat and poultry; raw or undercooked eggs.

Other suggestions

- Add extras such as vinegar, salt, lemon or lime juice to foods such as salads or the marinades for meat, as these additions can help reduce risks of contamination.
- It can also be a good idea to rinse raw meat such as chicken in salty water.
- Defrost food in the fridge, not at room temperature. Or leave it under running hot water or defrost carefully in the microwave.

Food poisoning

Symptoms of food poisoning may vary but are likely to include diarrhoea, stomach pain, nausea and vomiting, and sometimes fever, headache and muscle pains. Symptoms may also begin at varying times after eating the affected food, from a few hours to several days later.

If you are unfortunate enough to go down with food poisoning, do contact your doctor immediately and drink plenty of fluids – lemonade, flat cola, plain water and water with Dioralyte solution can all be helpful.

Safety with vitamin, mineral and other food supplements

Many people believe that over-the-counter 'natural' supplements, in whatever form, are both safe and efficacious. However, 'natural' does not necessarily equal 'safe'. Vitamins, tonics and other supplements are not subject to the rigorous testing that pharmaceutical drugs must undergo before they come on the market and can be safely prescribed. The food and drug authorities require years of research demonstrating efficacy as well as safety for use in humans before a pharmaceutical drug is approved for prescription. In contrast, the rules around vitamins, supplements and other health aids are relatively lax. In addition, food and drug authorities cannot withdraw an over-the-counter supplement unless it has been proven to cause serious harm, which in many cases can be difficult to demonstrate. This often means the claims made by the manufacturers and those recommending the products are at times exaggerated and rarely backed up by scientific trials or studies.

Some people argue that supplements are not drugs but just a food. Well, this is not really the case, as in most cases supplements are a very concentrated amount of some sort of chemical extracted from a food or other type of plant. Many drugs are simply active molecules which are derived from this type of chemical – aspirin being a classic example, as it was derived from willow bark.

The final thing I say to people is that if a supplement was as powerful or as potent as manufacturers often claim, you can bet your bottom dollar that one of the mega-pharmaceutical companies would have picked it up and trialled it as a drug!

Likewise, if any wonder supplement did exist, you could also be sure that your oncologist would be prescribing it as part of your anti-cancer treatment. The reason most oncologists do not recommend or prescribe such products is because there is not enough data behind them to ensure they are safe, effective and – most importantly – not going to interact with or limit the efficacy of your current treatment. It is not necessarily because oncologists do not support complementary or alternative medicine *per se*.

If you have heard of any over-the-counter products or supplements you would like to take, it is important to discuss this with your doctor, the pharmacist or the specialist nurse team. If you have already purchased the product, then you should take in the bottle or packet to ask about its suitability and the recommended dose. If you are taking some form of complementary remedy and are having side effects like wheezing, itching, numbness or tingling in your limbs, do contact your doctor or healthcare team and in the meanwhile start tapering off your dose of the product.

Of paramount concern is your safety and the certainty that the ingredients do not interfere with other aspects of your health. It's also vital that supplements don't affect the potency of cancer treatments. This is still an under-researched area, but definitely one in which it is best to err on the side of caution. A study in the *Journal of Clinical Oncology* looked at whether popular herbal remedies in the USA were likely to interact with cancer medication. The study suggested that, of the top-selling 15 products, nine may pose a risk of negative interactions, including ginseng, St John's wort, gingko and kava.

Safety with alternative diets

I'm sure you've heard plenty about wonder diets promoted as effective treatments for cancer. Some advise people with cancer to cut out dairy products or meat, or to live mostly on fresh juice, or to take mega-doses of some vitamin. Very often they go hand in hand with apparently irresistible endorsements from people who found that following them appeared dramatically to improve or even cure their cancer.

To the person struggling with cancer and the sometimes grim realities of treatment – fatigue, rushed appointments, hospital travel and parking charges, and so on – it is very understandable that such diets may appeal as being delightfully out of the clinical domain. They're something you can do for yourself, and as such completely under your control, with no unpleasant drugs and side effects. But while such diets may empower people with cancer, do they have any effect?

My own opinion, which I'm sure you'll have guessed by now, is that such diets are at best far more trouble than they're worth, and at worst potentially dangerous. As I said earlier in this book, now is not the time to be cutting major food groups out of your diet. To take just one simple example, some anti-cancer drugs have a bone-weakening effect – if you then give up dairy products, you run quite a risk of osteoporosis. On a more general level, very often such diets are far too restrictive, and can be not only tedious and expensive but positively harmful, as they can result in weight loss and malnutrition.

Diet in cancer causes a great deal of confusion, and perhaps nowhere more so than in this vexed area of 'wonder diets'. As I have stressed in this book, it is better to eat a balanced diet of the types of foods you enjoy than to put yourself through the mill, being a martyr to a horrible exclusive diet, just because you hope it is somehow good for you. If you do have any queries about alternative diets, or foods that you feel disagree with you, or food intolerances or allergies, again, do discuss them with a trained health professional. Because of the nutritional risks associated with these diets and at times the extra expense involved in purchasing supplements or 'special' drinks, you should discuss an interest in such approaches with your doctor or specialist before you hand over your credit card.

Probably more important than fad diets are the nutritional guidelines that have already been set up by years of rigorous research and thousands and thousands of well-accredited studies. (See page 16 for the key diet suggestions established by the work of the World Cancer Research Fund, and Chapter 10 for more on cancer prevention.)

We know that diet is a factor in around 30 per cent of cancers, making it second only to smoking as the most preventable cause of cancer (source: WCRF). The strongest links to some of the leading types of cancer are a higher than ideal body weight, lack of activity, too much alcohol and a poor intake of plant-based foods such as grains, fruits and vegetables. However, it is not possible to know exactly why one person ends up with cancer and others don't. When considering dietary factors it is important to realize that, in our current state of knowledge, many cases of cancer have no obvious causal factors behind them. While it makes sense to eat as well as you can, it also makes sense not to blame yourself or your previous diet for your illness.

9
Common questions

What foods should I avoid?

The short answer is simple: during treatment, avoid the foods that you can't tolerate or the foods that may make symptoms worse. For example, a very high-fibre or bulky diet is not the best for someone with a poor appetite who is also experiencing continuing bouts of diarrhoea. Otherwise there are no specific foods that need to be avoided unless your doctor tells you something different.

The starting point should be a typical well-balanced diet, with rather more emphasis on high quality protein foods, some grains, at least five to seven servings of fruits and vegetables and some limits on unhealthy fats and sugar.

But if this type of diet doesn't agree with you, or you are experiencing difficulties eating, it is up to you to work with your clinic and dietitian to find a more workable diet. For example, people with mouth sores may find that some fruits are too painful to eat. People with nausea and diarrhoea may find they just can't tolerate high-fibre breads and cereals. All this is nothing to worry about, as the treatment phase is just one window of the cancer journey and it doesn't last for ever. Nutrition is always about deciding on the highest priorities at the time, and then working the background diet around so it can support other longer-term health concerns.

Should I avoid dairy products if I have a hormonal cancer?

I've lost count of the number of people I've met who've given up eating dairy products when diagnosed with cancer, especially breast cancer. The notion that dairy products are deeply implicated in cancer development is pervasive and hard to shift, but really unfounded on the evidence!

Low-fat dairy foods are a good source of biologically rich protein and high in bio-available forms of calcium. Dairy also contains certain fats called conjugated linolenic acids which are a focus in health research. Extensive reviews of the scientific evidence have not found any strong links between dairy and breast cancer risks. There are also many benefits to including dairy foods in the diet.

Dairy foods have one of the highest quality sources of protein, far superior to soya equivalents. They are a source of an important amino acid, luecine, which is taken by many athletes to help with strength and muscle weight gain, and this is important during treatment. Dairy foods are also the best source of bio-available calcium, important for the bones, especially in those who are at risk of osteoporosis – which is all women who have been diagnosed at a pre-menopausal or menopausal age. The conjugated linolenic fats in milk also appear to actually help with weight loss as they promote fat excretion from the body.

The concerns around dairy products seem to relate to a belief that intensive farming methods increase exposure to hormones, and that somehow this definitely explains the breast cancer increases. This is unlikely to be the case in the UK, as bovine growth hormones are banned by EU food authorities and natural intakes due to use of pregnant bovines are minute. Furthermore, these substances are proteins and are broken down in the acidic environment of the stomach, so actual amounts that might be absorbed are negligible, certainly compared to amounts taken in from hormone sources such as contraceptive pills.

Other theories have stemmed from population studies comparing Western and Asian cultures (i.e. US and Japanese women), which broadly examined breast cancer rates along with a spectrum of lifestyle and diet differences. One of the reasons proposed for the higher rate of breast cancer in Western women was the dairy intake. However, there are so many more differences between these populations, including levels of fat intake, energy intake, fish intake, activity, genetics and alcohol intake. There are also different approaches to the levels of routine screening, and intervention and record-keeping across different regions in Asia varies enormously. These, along with many more factors, could equally be pinpointed as possible causes.

Finally and importantly, a number of case-controlled studies have not found any link; in fact, at this point the research is actually leaning towards a lower risk in individuals who are higher dairy consumers (Harvie and Ackermann 2006).

If you are intolerant to lactose – which is common with any treatment that may affect the gut lining – it may be worth trying a lactose-free milk. This is available in the supermarket chill section alongside the regular milks. People who have a degree of lactose intolerance also tend to manage some cheese and small amounts of yoghurt. Cottage cheese is a whey-rich protein source, and some research indicates that whey protein again may be more beneficial to weight and muscle gain.

Does sugar feed cancer? Should I avoid sugar if I have cancer?

No!!!

This is one of the most commonly asked questions, and I have met many people who have tried to cut sugar out of their diet. However, what needs to be understood is that sugar is a type of carbohydrate. Carbohydrates are an important energy food, and every cell in the body requires glucose or sugar to function. For example, the brain wholly and solely uses glucose or sugar to keep it functioning. A drop in blood sugar can cause feelings of fatigue, dizziness and faintness.

When you eat any kind of carbohydrate (found in desserts, sweetened drinks, fruits, milk, grains and starchy vegetables), the body breaks those carbohydrates down into a range of simple sugars, which are then converted into glucose to be taken into the cells. Therefore, the idea that sugar somehow 'feeds' cancer is neither useful nor correct – sugar, as a form of carbohydrate, feeds every cell in our bodies.

However, what is important to understand is that there are different types or quality grades of carbohydrate foods. There are the wholesome grain type foods, fruits, vegetables and dairy foods which can move more slowly (slow-release or low GI type carbohydrates) and then there are those which are more processed, mixed with higher-calorie, higher-fat snack food type ingredients and typically these are absorbed quite quickly (high GI or fast-release types).

When our diet includes more of the fast-release or high GI types (refined or more processed carbohydrate foods) this requires the body to produce more of the hormone insulin. Insulin is needed to enable the cells to take up glucose from the blood into the muscle cells. However, several spikes of insulin across the day could be a risk factor for cancer as well as weight gain. (Insulin is a growth hormone and promotes fat storage.) The slower-release carbohydrate foods (grains, dairy, colder weather fruits and vegetables) are absorbed and used in the body over two or three hours and do not require such a rapid insulin response (lower levels), as the slower release means that the blood sugar levels do not spike at such a high level. The body is always working to keep our blood sugar levels within a normal ideal range. A rapid rise in blood sugar means the body responds in a panic and produces larger amounts of insulin. A gradual and more level rise in the blood sugar enables the body to have more time to process the sugar and it doesn't result in excessive amounts of insulin floating around the system.

For an all-round balanced diet, it is best to get your energy needs met by a range of lower GI carbohydrates such as vegetables, fruit, wholegrains and legumes (beans). However, at the same time there is no need to become fanatical about this – sugar is not like some kind of deadly poison. If you fancy a little bit of luxury chocolate or a slice of delicious home-baked carrot cake, have it. Gosh, you are in treatment for cancer and you should also enjoy your food!

One other point to bear in mind is that you can't always judge your carbohydrate needs in cancer by your normal carbohydrate needs. This is a complex area, and one where the individual component in cancer cases must be borne in mind. Many people find that the toll of the illness and the impact the treatments have on the body compromise its nutrient stores. Because of the extra load caused by the cancer growing in the body, the treatment side effects and sometimes a wasting effect (cachexia), there may be a need for extra calories, and some extra carbohydrate foods can help out here. So, when considering your overall carbohydrate intake, again do discuss your individual needs with your doctor or dietitian if necessary.

Can I drink alcohol?

Let me say straight out that a little of what you fancy is no bad thing here. A small glass of wine or sherry before a meal can help stimulate your appetite and make a meal a more relaxed and enjoyable occasion.

The emphasis, however, is on 'small'. Alcohol has been linked with an increased risk of developing some types of cancer. In particular, some studies have shown that as little as three units a day can increase the risk of oesophagus, mouth, throat, breast and bowel cancers. As alcohol is high in calories, it may also be a risk factor if it contributes to being overweight.

Current sensible drinking guidelines recommend that:

- men drink no more than two units of alcohol per day, or 14 per week;
- women drink no more than one unit per day, or 7 per week.

One unit of alcohol is the equivalent of a small glass of wine (125 ml), half a pint of standard strength beer, cider or lager, or a single measure (25 ml) of a standard-strength spirit.

Drinking large quantities of alcohol in one session (binge drinking) is thought to be worse for your health than drinking a small amount each day. It is also recommended that people have one or two non-drinking days each week.

If you are taking any medicines, check with your doctor or pharmacist that you may drink alcohol.

Should I eat only organic foods?

The term 'organic' is used to describe foods grown without pesticides or herbicides. Organic foods have on occasions been found to be higher in vitamin C and lower in nitrates; however, the comparisons are variable. Farmers who produce organic produce may also help to protect the environment. However, other farmers do this as well but may not have gone to the trouble and expense of obtaining certification.

What is more important than whether the food is organic are the types and amounts of different foods consumed. You are better off eating a corn cob that isn't organic than eating organic French fries! Eating the recommended servings of fruit and vegetables will benefit your health whether they are organic or not. There is no current evidence to suggest that other organic produce can help reduce the risk of cancer.

Do wash all non-organic fruits and vegetables thoroughly before they are consumed to remove any traces of pesticides.

Should I stop eating meat?

While it does appear that a diet high in fruit and vegetables is more protective against cancer, during treatment high protein foods such as lean meat and dairy provide your body with more of the important build-up nutrients that it needs for repair, recovery and energy.

I would recommend that you do not cut out red meat or the like during the treatment. However, try to ensure that the meat you choose is of a high quality and is purchased from a reputable farmer.

After the treatment period, the WCRF UK cancer prevention guidelines recommend an intake of around 500 g of cooked meat per week (or 700 g raw). This includes beef, pork and lamb.

In general it is best to avoid processed meat such as processed ham, bacon, frankfurters, salami and some sausages. Cancer-causing substances (carcinogens) can be formed when red meat is preserved by smoking, curing or salting, or by the addition of preservatives. These substances can damage cells in the body, leading to the development of cancer. Having said that, I would not worry too much during the treatment phase if you are feeling like these sorts of foods on occasions.

Will eating less fat lower my risk of cancer recurrence?

Although there is no evidence of a direct link between fat intake and an increased cancer risk, evidence suggests that a high-fat diet may increase the risk of breast cancer (in post-menopausal women) and lung cancer, and diets high in animal or saturated fat may increase the risk for colorectal cancer. As high fat consumption can contribute to obesity, and obesity is a strong risk factor for several cancers, you should limit your intake of high-fat foods. This is an important concern if you have a cancer which is associated with weight gain.

Should I juice vegetables and fruit?

On the whole it is much better to eat whole fruit and vegetables than to juice them, because they contain fibre as well as lower amounts of sugar. Some of the natural goodness may be lost in juicing, too, as some vitamins deteriorate quickly once exposed to air, light or knife damage. However, during the treatment it may be easier for you to include your fruit and vegetables as a juice or a smoothie. If you can, try to consume your juice soon after preparation.

If you are trying to contain your weight, you need to remember that juices are much higher in calories than whole vegetables or fruit, which can be a problem if you over-consume.

Is soy good if I have had breast cancer?

As part of a healthy diet, a moderate intake of soya foods (such as soya milk, tofu, etc.) is considered perfectly acceptable.

However, there is no evidence that soy or phyto-oestrogen supplements prevent or cure any form of cancer. Some studies have indicated that in supplement form phyto-oestrogens may in fact stimulate existing tumour growth and antagonize the effects of some cancer treatment. Therefore soy or phyto-oestrogen supplements should not be taken.

What should I do if the person I am caring for does not want to eat and is losing weight?

As I've said earlier in this book, there can be a fine line between tempting someone's appetite and pushing them to eat, especially when your loved one with cancer genuinely has no appetite. If your best efforts don't work, do speak to the doctor. Report the weight loss – how much, and over what period – and try and keep a diary of what food has been consumed. Have a look at the tips for tempting a flagging appetite on page 102. Meanwhile, things to try include:

- Provide smaller portions and serve on a tray nicely presented with a napkin and maybe a flower in a vase.
- Think in terms of a child's tea party, with a range of tempting nibbles such as tiny egg and cress sandwiches without crusts, small biscuits (such as Iced Gems), smoked salmon and cream cheese on savoury cheese biscuits, small home-made scones with butter and jam, roasted chicken breast with a tiny portion of home-made chips, individual steak and kidney puddings (available from the chill section of many supermarkets if you don't want to cook them yourself).
- Regularly offer snacks such as milkshakes (add a dollop of ice cream) and Twiglets; a small glass of Guinness with a cheese sandwich; an individual serving of apricot crumble (make at home with dried or tinned apricots).
- Get together a range of TV snacks to nibble while viewing, such as fingers of toast and butter or Marmite toast, popcorn, thick-cut or home-made crisps, pieces of good quality chocolate, speciality bread such as Turkish or corn chips with a lovely dip such as guacamole, cream cheese or hummus; thin slices of hard speciality cheese such as Manchego (traditionally eaten with quince preserve, but a good quality digestive biscuit and/or grapes might be easier and less rich!).

Help! I'm putting *on* weight during treatment – what can I do?

Historically, much of the attention given to nutrition during cancer treatments has been very focused on building up and staying strong during treatment. I suspect this is because as dietitians we are often asked to meet people who are having problems eating and whose nutritional health is in decline. Often, those who are gaining weight are not flagged and advised on nutrition, until in desperation they plead with their doctors for some help or guidance.

However, it also needs to be emphasized that not all people lose weight, and in fact many people find that they do gain weight. Quite often, this weight gain jumps up quickly to more than 5–10 kg (11–22 lb) throughout the treatment period. Do discuss your weight with your medical team, but meanwhile here are some tips.

The top ten tips for weight management during treatment

1 Eat small, regular meals based around the healthy eating guidelines (see <www.nhs.uk/Livewell/Goodfood/Pages/eight-tips-healthy-eating.aspx>). In addition to the UK healthy eating guidelines, I like the plate model used to depict healthy eating in the USA; visit ≤www.choosemyplate.gov> and refer to the 2010 US dietary guidelines.

2 Include extra protein, both at mealtimes and as a snack. For example, some tuna, eggs, lean meat, chicken, other fish, low-fat dairy foods, etc.

3 Choose small amounts of wholegrain or lower GI type cereal foods as part of each meal, for example brown rice, pasta, grain-based bread, natural muesli, whole or pinhead oats, oat cakes, malt loaf.

4 Bulk up with extra vegetables, e.g. cabbage in stir-fries, corn, dark leafy vegetables.

5 Ensure you are well hydrated. In addition to water, include sugar-free squash or herbal or chai type teas.

6 Keep being as active as you can. Try gentle exercise classes; walk when you can; try to include some light weights sessions if appropriate. Ideally, keep up 30–45 minutes of exercise or activity a day.

7 Write down what you eat or take a couple of days' worth of food pictures with a phone or digital camera. A daily record helps identify times or binge patterns which jeopardize your efforts to stay at your ideal weight.

8 Don't let yourself get hungry. If you miss meals or skimp, it is likely you will find yourself very hungry and end up wanting to binge or gorge at the next mealtime.

9 Trim extra calories where you can, either by limiting added fats and sugars or by containing portion sizes.

10 Go for quality, not quantity. Everyone enjoys a treat, especially when you are in treatment. Don't deprive yourself, but choose something that will give you a real lift. A tasty piece of tropical fruit, some ruby red strawberries, a juicy orange, a piece of dark, quality chocolate, a small piece of delicious home-made cake, honey sourced from local bees on some appetizing baked sourdough, some Scottish smoked salmon, a piece of pungent (pasteurized) cheese from a speciality shop, a flavoursome Italian meal – you get the picture.

10

After treatment: a word on healthy eating and cancer prevention

This is a very important topic, although mostly beyond the scope of this book, which focuses on the dietary priorities around the treatment phase of having cancer. However, one thing to emphasize here is that there is a difference between eating to prevent cancer and eating when you are in treatment for cancer.

Research has shown that a healthy weight, being active and plant-based dietary approaches may help prevent around 30 per cent of cancers, but once you actually have the disease it is still not clear to what extent diet can influence its progress or risk of recurrence. This is a growing area of research and more scientific studies are needed before we can fully understand the role of diet and lifestyle in the prevention of cancer after recovery from treatments for the disease.

Hence at this time the recommendations for eating well and being active are that, after treatment for cancer, people should follow the primary cancer prevention guidelines.

WCRF UK's recommendations for cancer prevention

1 Be as lean as possible without becoming underweight.
2 Be physically active for at least 30 minutes every day.
3 Avoid sugary drinks and limit consumption of energy-dense foods (particularly processed foods high in added sugar, or low in fibre, or high in fat).
4 Eat more of a variety of vegetables, fruits, wholegrains and pulses such as beans.
5 Limit consumption of red meats (such as beef, pork and lamb) and avoid processed meats.

6 If consumed at all, limit alcoholic drinks to two a day for men and one a day for women.

7 Limit consumption of salty foods and food processed with salt (sodium).

8 Don't use supplements to protect against cancer.

9 It is best for mothers to breastfeed exclusively for up to six months and then add other liquids and foods.

10 After treatment, cancer survivors should follow the general recommendations for cancer prevention.

And always remember – do not smoke or chew tobacco.

Please be aware that these guidelines will not be suitable for everyone after treatment. If you are underweight, have experienced significant weight loss, have had surgery affecting your digestive system, have swallowing difficulties or have bowel problems or any other difficulties eating a normal diet, you should ask your doctor, dietitian or specialist nurse if these recommendations are suitable for you.

Diet and cancer prevention

The guidelines are also general guidelines for cancer prevention. However, the different types of cancer can all be influenced by different dietary factors. You can find out more about factors which either have no impact or can increase or decrease the risk of some of the dietary-related cancers from the WCRF/AICR's Expert Report, *Food, Nutrition, Physical Activity, and the Prevention of Cancer: a global perspective*. Amendments and updates are constantly being made as we continue to gather more research around diet, exercise and cancer prevention.

Although some of the terms may not be familiar to you, it gives an idea of the range and depth of the scientific research that went into producing the Report. Visit <www.dietandcancerreport.org> to find out more about it.

I also invite you to download or order a booklet I wrote with WCRF, *Eating Well and Being Active Following Cancer Treatment*. It provides more detail on the Report and guidelines for healthy lifestyle approaches to help reduce cancer risks after treatment. It is available for free from <http://www.wcrf-uk.org/PDFs/ EatingWellBeingActive.pdf> or the WCRF (see Useful addresses).

The following topic is one I like to discuss with the people attending the nutrition presentation in our cancer survivor programme.

Working with more 'superfoods' in your diet

You will often hear that this food or that is the latest superfood, or that one food is better or has more super-antioxidant powers than another. Turmeric is claimed to be a better spice than cumin. The gogi berry is apparently better than the pomegranate, and of course dark chocolate and red wine have been given the green light. In actual fact I am quite sick of hearing about the latest and greatest superfood – and really there is no such thing, as variety is what it is all about.

However, across the cancer research world there has been continuing interest in a particular group of food chemicals called the phytochemicals. Scientists have been working to unravel the mechanisms and potential therapeutic benefits of many of these potent phytochemicals, which occur naturally in plant foods, to determine whether they have a role in cancer prevention and other health problems.

This is not an easy task as there are over 100,000 different phytochemicals in plant foods including fruits, vegetables, nuts, seeds, pulses and wholegrain cereal foods. There can also be quite wide variations between concentrations according to the season, the plant variety, the ripeness of the food and whether the phytochemicals exert their effects individually or synergistically – in other words, do combinations work together to exert an overall greater benefit?

One group of French researchers have tried to narrow the field somewhat and have started looking at one group of these phytochemicals, called polyphenols. Polyphenols have been an area of interest around cancer research for some time: there have been over 6,000 studies on polyphenols and cancer.

What is helpful to us practically minded folk is that this French research has measured and listed for us the top 100 polyphenol-rich foods. Using a method which is more advanced than those used previously, they have put together the Phenol Explorer database <http://www.phenol-explorer.eu/>.

Introducing the polyphenols

Polyphenols are a large class of compounds found in plants. They help defend against attack by insects and give plants their colour. From our point of view, they are valuable because they are some of the most potent antioxidants available. They have a particular chemical compound structure characterized by the presence of at least one 'phenol' unit and so are also referred to as phenolics. 'Poly' means 'many' and 'polyphenols' simply indicates large numbers of these compounds grouped together. While no one can be expected to remember them all – there are over 4,000 different polyphenol compounds – it is good to know that they are on your side and act as powerful antioxidants that can neutralize free radicals, reduce inflammation and slow tumour growth.

A good way of knowing whether they might be in your food is that these polyphenols are the chemicals that give the bite or astringency to foods. You'll notice it in tea that's brewed too strong (the compound once called tannin) and in the 'greenish' flavour of extra-virgin olive oil or the back palate of red wine. Anything that makes your mouth pucker a little generally contains polyphenols.

Although there are thousands of polyphenols, a few examples include: resveratrol, found in red wine; capsaicin, found in chilli and paprika; thymol, found in thyme; cinnamic acid, found in cinnamon; and rosmarinic acid, found in rosemary, thyme, oregano, sage and peppermint (remember my push for herbs and spices?).

The new top 100

The Phenol Explorer database has summarized polyphenols in two top 100 lists – the first gives the richest 100 foods by concentration, while the second has foods ranked by their content per serving. The lists show you the best foods and beverages that provide more than 1 mg of total polyphenols per serving.

They range from 15,000 mg per 100 g for cloves down to a tiny 10 mg per 100ml for rosé wine. Many spices and dried herbs appear on the 'per 100 g' list but not on the 'per serving' list as their serving size is so small (usually less than a gram or a pinch), although this richness is another good reason to remember to try to use them to add more flavour to your foods.

Tea, on the other hand is ranked only 52 (black) and 54 (green) on the 'per 100 g' list but makes it to 16 and 17 in the 'per serving' list, as we drink sizeable quantities (200 ml/7 oz in a cup); for many people tea will be their main source of polyphenols.

So while this information is helpful and interesting, it needs to be emphasized that it is not about paying inflated prices for the latest superfoods, but about jazzing up meals with some top-up tastes, more colour and spice, and more variety from the thousands of these potent health-supporting nutrients.

Here are a few more ideas for how you can do this. Remember, it means aiming for lots of colours of fruits, vegetables, nuts, seeds and wholegrain cereals, and it is very easy to open a can of pulses to add to a salad or the family stew.

Incorporating more plant foods rich in polyphenols into your diet

Try to add a little more of the following:

- Spices: cloves, star anise, capers, curry powder, ginger, cumin, cinnamon, turmeric.
- Herbs (including dried): peppermint, oregano, sage, rosemary, thyme, basil, lemon verbena, parsley, marjoram, coriander.
- Seeds: flaxseeds, celery seeds.
- Nuts: chestnuts, hazelnuts, pecans, almonds, walnuts, pine nuts.
- Bread: rye, wholegrain wheat flour, soy and linseed breads (Vogel).
- Olives: black olives, green olives.
- Vegetables: globe artichokes, spinach, red chicory, green chicory, red onions, spinach, broccoli, curly endive, peppers, potatoes, pulses, carrots.
- Dark berries: black chokeberry, elderberry, blueberry, plum, cherry, blackcurrant, blackberry, strawberry, raspberry, prune, black grapes, redcurrants.
- Fruit other than berries: apples and apple juice, nectarines, pomegranates and pomegranate juice, peaches, grapefruit juice, blood oranges and blood orange juice, lemon juice, lime juice, apricots, quinces, grapes, prunes, pears.
- Oils: extra-virgin olive oil, rapeseed (canola) oil.
- Beverages and extras: filter coffee, green tea, black tea, red wine (in moderation), cocoa beverages with milk, dark chocolate, soya tofu, soya milk and yoghurt.

Remember, this is a fast-moving science and not all foods have been measured yet. The researchers also mention the following as worth keeping in mind:

- Lentils, dried oregano, dried summer savoury, dried bay leaves, dried camomile, dried coriander, fenugreek, dried winter savoury, pistachio, hyssop, red Swiss chard leaves, dried dill, raisins, black pepper, fresh peppermint, figs, fresh lemon balm, fenugreek seed, tarragon.

Energize yourself with some 'superfood' suggestions

Remember, if you are having trouble eating or swallowing, to adjust the texture of the food using a hand-held blender.

Breakfast
- Orange, cut into quarters
- Bowl of whole oats with an added seed and berry mix, a topping of fresh berries, a sprinkle of cinnamon and skimmed or soya milk
- Cup of tea.

Lunch
- Vegetable soup (try beetroot, carrot, minestrone, lentil and chard, etc.)
- Salmon, avocado and baby spinach salad with baby tomatoes, with a vinaigrette dressing made with flaxseed oil, garlic, chopped parsley, coriander and lemon juice
- Soy and linseed thick toast or wholegrain pitta bread.

Dinner
- Grilled lean lamb cutlets or chicken with basil pesto sauce, broccoli, asparagus, carrots
- Small serving of brown rice or baby or new potatoes
- Low-fat berry yoghurt with extra fresh blueberries (drizzle melted dark chocolate for a treat).

Snacks
- Apple, oat and flaxseed muffin
- Handful of nuts mixed with dried raisins and organic apricots

- Home-made berry smoothie (make with fresh or frozen berries)
- Fresh fruit
- Crackers
- Slice of malt loaf or fruit bread.

Table 10.1 lists some simple ideas for bringing more phytonutrients into your day.

Learning to cook for enjoyment and health

The more you experiment with cooking, the better and more confident you will become. This gives you more ability not only to enjoy your old favourites, but also to make small changes that will improve taste and flavour as well as the contribution they can make towards your health.

If you have not been a regular cook, learning may seem difficult at first. However, it is exactly like trying to learn a new sport or language – it feels uncomfortable or impossible to start with, but the more you practise the better you become.

Part of learning to cook is to become familiar with a wide range of fresh and interesting ingredients. Try your local farmers' market, fishmonger or speciality food outlets. Talk to the suppliers and try to learn more about food and its ingredients. It can also be helpful to have good equipment (non-stick frying pan, electric griller, wok, microwave, food processor, hand-held blender, oven rack, baking paper) and a good set of knives.

It is important not to be afraid to make changes to the way you prepare many of the traditional dishes you may have cooked.

Hints for adapting recipes

- Reduce the butter, oil or cream that you add to recipes. Usually the same results can be achieved by using a fraction of the original quantities, particularly in older-style recipes. Other substitutes can include low-fat yoghurt, ricotta cheese or evaporated skimmed milk.
- Instead of frying in oil or butter, cook basic ingredients such as onion or garlic in water. This is just a lower-fat approach to cooking. For example, if you are making a soup it is fine to cook the onions and garlic in water instead of oil.

Table 10.1 Some simple ideas for bringing more phytonutrients into your day

Swap the regulars . . .	. . . for some of these alternatives or additions
Iceberg lettuce	Darker lettuce such as mignonette, baby spinach, rocket, red cabbage, parsley (try tabouli), chervil leaves
Potato	Sweet potato, pumpkin, chick peas, lentils, aubergines, parsnip, baby potatoes, corn, beetroot (mix in spices like nutmeg)
Green beans	Spinach, bok choy, peas, chard, cabbage
Pears and apples	Oranges, mandarins, grapefruit, tangelo, berries, kiwi fruit, mango, pawpaw, pomegranate, pineapple (add cloves, cinnamon, star anise, mint)
Potato crisps	Mixed nuts, salted cashews, almonds, walnuts
White fish fillets	Atlantic salmon, fresh tuna, canned salmon, canned sardines, swordfish
Puffed or flaked cereal	Oat-based cereal (muesli, rolled oats, oat and fruit flakes) or sprinkle a tablespoon of ground flax or linseed or rice bran over your favourite cereal
Ice cream	Thick low-fat Greek yoghurt topped with cinnamon (or other mixed spices) and honey, low-fat soya or custard
Salt	Sage, coriander, lemon juice, sherry vinegar, ginger, cumin, black pepper, basil, chilli

- Drain meat if cooking in a frying pan. For example, if you are cooking a bolognese sauce you should strain the meat to allow the fat to drip away after browning.
- Switch to low-salt varieties, and instead of adding salt to your cooking learn to appreciate the tastes of fresh herbs, lemon and garlic.
- Readjust the portions of meat to vegetables in your recipes. Allow a small palm-sized portion of meat per person and bulk up with more vegetables, legumes such as lentils, chickpeas, barley, rice or pasta. Small canned varieties of beans are a quick and easy way to add legumes to your cooking.

- Trim all the fat off the meat you do eat. Take the skin off the chicken and trim all visible fat off meat; roast on a rack.
- Filo pastry can be used to make a quiche or pie instead of the more traditional types of pastry.
- Try oil-free bastes or marinades.
- Popcorn can be cooked in the microwave and eaten unbuttered.
- If you are baking, try to cut the butter or margarine by one-third. Add some extra fruit such as a mix of dried or mashed fresh fruit, e.g. mango or banana can be folded into a cake mixture.
- Try not to add sugar to recipes. Sweeten with stewed fresh fruit or try vanilla essence.
- Heavy sauces are out these days. Instead of a gravy or cream-based sauce, try a lighter jus or just splash on some good quality balsamic vinegar.

Conclusion

One of the most humbling experiences I can share is when I meet up with a group of our patients who are either at an active stage or towards the end of their cancer treatment experiences. These people have taken time out to attend one of our group sessions on a range of topics; the one I talk on is nutrition, and I feel privileged to share their stories and experiences. They come to help find answers to their questions, and at times to find their way forward or out of a hole, and the friendship and support they share with each other is something beyond special.

However, when it comes to nutrition many of the experiences people share are those that seemed to have knocked them sideways or confused them, and often they have grabbed the wrong end of the stick. Many of the food ideals that have been reinvented to help them cope are negative or bewildering and can almost pull them away from the balance, tastes and health factors which count. Some people admit to being genuinely scared about what foods they should eat; they are unsure which way to turn or how now to fill their trolley; sometimes they don't want to go out at all. There is a constant barrage of questions about this pill or that potion.

I totally understand why people feel like this: they are desperate and just want to do whatever they can to help, at no matter what cost. So I start our session by throwing them into what I hope is a more indulgent food world and by sharing with them some experiences, the science, the facts and as much practical know-how as I can, to show them a better way to fit it all in.

As soon as they are seated and we have introduced the session, I get the participants to close their eyes, take a few deep breaths and think back to a time (hopefully lots of times) when they felt elated with a lively food experience – a special meal, great food or a memory of spending time luxuriating over courses with family, friends or people who inspire.

When I think back over my own food memories, I remember my time travelling around the UK and across Europe and, more recently, travels in and around Asia, all based on earlier experiences in my home town of Sydney, Australia. I think of freshly caught fish, barbecue-grilled, accompanied by a crisp salad with the juiciest red tomatoes that explode with flavour; olives; a lemon, balsamic vinegar and extra virgin olive oil dressing at a beach café in southern Italy; the juiciest steak cooked at our table by a chef restaurant owner of 30 years; diving into paper-wrapped fish and chips while trying to warm up after a day at a Devon beach; the cheese plate selected by the young passionate waiter, while we lounged in front of a roaring fire in a French ski hut restaurant with our oldest friends; the surprise tastes of a degustation menu (a menu with small portions of unusual dishes for testing) introduced with some French champagne and lingered over with old friends in a three-star organic farm restaurant; designing and serving a five-course meal at my home for a school charity auction; the marinated lamb shoulder on the barbecue at a friend's waterfront home on the Costa Brava in Spain.

But it doesn't have to be linked with holidays: there's meeting a friend for a coffee brewed with selected coffee beans; creamy scrambled eggs on sourdough toast at a favourite local café; strolling around the local farmers' market buying dirt-covered baby and sweet potatoes, dark green broccoli, real beetroots freshly dug, honey from a hive at the local park, a homemade cottage pie, fresh fish, succulent lamb chops and homemade relishes that bite; a pub lunch at the end of a long country walk, and a meal on the fire at the campsite with friends.

And then the pick-your-own fields where the children wonder at the fruit and vegetables growing, then filling the buckets with strawberries, beans, cobs of corn, juicy red apples, raspberries . . . and then working out what to cook up with them; running a cooking programme at my children's school, making fresh pasta and using a pasta-cutting machine, then picking fresh basil leaves to make a pesto recipe worked up by an Italian mother . . .

Many of the people I have worked with, during their treatment stage and beyond, have become friends and a constant source of inspiration. I more than understand that this is not an easy time, and my role is to try and help these people who inspire me and who I call my friends, and now, I hope, the people who read this book, to understand that food for all its important health and essential nourishing properties has a bigger role, which is one that gives passage to life's celebrations, many special times, moments and more. When eating is not easy or possible, then nutrition and food must be about being creative and still trying to capture the experiences and time spent together at a table, on a picnic rug, by the fire or walking in and around markets and speciality food or farm shops.

Wherever your cancer journey takes you, I urge you not only to aim for good nutrition, but to search recipe sites and local restaurant reviews and to flick through colourful cookbooks. Always try to be positive about food and nutrition, to sit around the family table, to make eating celebratory and to progress with more and more foods and experiences that will boost, build and help to take you forward.

At the same time, consider how your body needs to be nourished: ensure you either get in the top-ups or contain eating if you need to. Work hard to hold your shape close to your ideal, and seek guidance if you know that things do not seem right.

The final summary

Engaging with nutrition in cancer treatments and beyond should aim to provide:

1 The health benefits – aim for what is most pertinent to your current treatment needs, and then beyond.
2 A palate of colour – the appearance of a meal is the first invitation to eat, and the more colour, the more ingredients which can be incorporated: red and blue fruits, green leafy veg, grated carrots, mashed sweet potatoes, etc. The eye will always eat first, and the more colour, the more exciting the meal.
3 Textures and temperature – work with a combination of silky and, if possible, lots of crunch. Warm, temperate and refreshingly cool can all help a tormented mouth.
4 Taste – find the delicate balance your taste buds need between sweet and savoury, salty and bitter. This is described in Eastern cuisines as the ying and the yang of food. You need to establish what works best for you.
5 Umami – an after-taste experience which will be a feeling in the body or an after-taste explosion in the mouth.

There will be many pieces in the jigsaw of your cancer journey experience, and at times others will be more important than the nutrition piece *per se*. However, I hope that, by actively engaging with nutrition using the best approach you can, good eating, delicious food or tastes, the experiences around food times, the sourcing of exciting or comforting ingredients and produce will give you more pleasure than you could ever have imagined. I also hope that this positive relationship with food will keep you going towards the stage of beating cancer and beyond.

Appendix
Drink and meal supplements

Table A.1 Nutritional supplement range

Nutrition product manufacturers' contact information	Customer care number and website	Complete nutrition range energy 1.5 kcal/*–2 kcal	Nutritionally balanced range Powdered supplement drinks, soups	Protein powders and gels	Energy powders and liquids	Concentrated energy drinks Energy approx. 3 kcal/ml
Abbott Nutrition Abbott House Vanwall Business Park Vanwall Road Maidenhead Berkshire SL6 4XE	0800 252882 www.abbott nutrition.co.uk	Ensure Plus range • Milkshake-like * (banana, chocolate, vanilla, coffee, caramel, blackcurrant, neutral, peach, coffee, raspberry, strawberry) • Juice * (apple, fruit punch, lemon and lime, strawberry, orange, peach) • Yoghurt * (orange burst, orchard peach, pineapple twist and strawberry swirl) • Added fibre * (raspberry, chocolate, vanilla, banana, strawberry, fruits of the forest) • Ensure TwoCal (banana, neutral, strawberry, vanilla) • Puddings (banana, chocolate and vanilla flavours) • Prosure: 1.5 kcal/ml specialist feed with omega-3 fatty acids, antioxidants and fibre	Enshake (banana, chocolate, strawberry and vanilla)		Polycose powder	

Company	Contact	Products		
Nutricia Ltd, White Horse Business Park, Newmarket Avenue, Trowbridge, Wiltshire BA14 0XQ	01225 711677 www.nutricia.co.uk	Fortisip range • Milkshake-like * Scandishake (neutral, vanilla, chocolate, toffee, banana, orange, strawberry, tropical) • Juice * with added fibre (orange, strawberry, banana, vanilla and chocolate) • Yoghurt (raspberry, peach and orange, vanilla and lemon) • Puddings (Forticreme/Forticreme Complete) * • Savoury soup style with added fibre (chicken and tomato) • Forticare: 1.6 kcal/ml specialist feed with omega-3 fatty acids, antioxidants and fibre	Protifar	Maxijul powder Polycal powder Polycal liquid
Nestlé HealthCare Nutrition St George's House Croydon Surrey CR9 1NR	00800 6887 4846 www.nestlenutrition.co.uk	Resource Drink range • Resource Energy * (apricot, chocolate, strawberry/raspberry, banana, coffee, vanilla) • Resource Fruit Juice * (apple, orange, pear–cherry, raspberry–blackcurrant) • Resource Energy Dessert • Resource (2 kcal/ml) + Fibre (vanilla, summer fruits, strawberry, apricot, neutral, coffee) Build-up shakes (strawberry, chocolate, vanilla, banana) Build-up soups (chicken, potato and leek, tomato, vegetable)		Caloreen powder

Nutrition product manufacturers' contact information	Customer care number and website	Complete nutrition range energy 1.5 kcal*–2 kcal	Nutritionally balanced range Powdered supplement drinks, soups	Protein powders and gels	Energy powders and liquids	Concentrated energy drinks Energy approx. 3 kcal/ml
Fresenius Kabi Ltd Cestrian Court Eastgate Way Manor Park Runcorn Cheshire WA7 1NT	01928 533533 www2.fresenius-kabi.co.uk	Fresubin Energy Drink range • Milkshake-like (chocolate, neutral, vanilla, banana, strawberry, cappuccino) • Juice-like (tropical fruits, lemon, blackcurrant) • Fresubin Jucy (apple, orange, blackcurrant, cherry, pineapple; whey protein, suitable for fat malabsorption) • Added fibre (chocolate, vanilla, strawberry, banana, caramel, cherry) • Yocreme (125 g pot): available in five flavours (neutral, lemon, apricot–peach, raspberry, biscuit)			Calshake powder	Fresubin: 5 kcal/ml 3–4 shots per day provide 450–600 kcal
Vitaflo International Ltd Suite 1.11 South Harrington Building 128 Sefton Street Brunswick Business Park Liverpool L3 4BQ	0151 7099020 www.vitaflo.co.uk	• Supportan: 1.5 kcal/ml specialist feed with omega-3 fatty acids, antioxidants and fibre		Vitapro powder	Vitajoule powder	Pro-Cal shots

Complan Foods Nutricia Ltd (see page 147)	0845 6003170 www.complan.com	Complan Shakes (vanilla, chocolate, strawberry, banana)		
SHS International Ltd 100 Wavertree Boulevard Liverpool L7 9PT	0151 2288161 www.nutricia.co.uk	Max Pro Max-Sorb (whey-protein based)	Maxi Joule powder and liquid	Calogen/Calogen Extra (4 kcal/ml)
Nutrinovo Ltd 6 Cowper Road River Kent CT17 0PF	01304 829068 www.nutrinovo.com	Liquid Prosource – 10 g protein, 100 kcal per 30 ml serving (neutral, orange creme, citrus berry)		

Useful addresses

Reaching out for extra help, guidance and support

In the UK there are many groups and charities who will reach out to you with extra information, along with the support and additional guidance you may need. Cancer is not something to go through on your own; there will be people available to talk to, meet up with and discuss the issues with. In addition, most groups have a range of booklets, as well as their own websites, which can be useful as reminders of particular concerns or sources of information about areas you might like to explore further.

Organizations that can give you extra advice on nutrition

Breast Cancer Haven
(London Haven)
Effie Road
London SW6 1TB
Tel.: 020 7384 0099
Website: www.breastcancerhaven.org.uk

There are also Havens in Hereford (01432 361061) and Leeds (0113 284 7829). All the Havens provide a wide range of therapies, completely free of charge, which help people to deal with the physical and emotional side effects of breast cancer. Specialist nurses and experts in nutrition, exercise and emotional support provide tailor-made programmes for every person who comes through their doors. Their outreach programme has been specially developed for people who can't get to Havens so they can benefit from the organization's unique care in the comfort of their own home.

British Dietetic Association (BDA)
Fifth Floor, Charles House
148–9 Great Charles Street Queensway
Birmingham B3 3HT
Tel.: 0121 200 8080
Website: www.bda.uk.com

The BDA has a number of food fact sheets on its website which provide reviews on nutrition.

British Nutrition Foundation
High Holborn House
52–54 High Holborn
London WC1V 6RQ
Tel.: 020 7404 6504
Website: www.nutrition.org.uk

The British Nutrition Foundation is a scientific charity which promotes the wellbeing of the population by the impartial interpretation and effective dissemination of nutrition knowledge and advice based on scientific evidence. It provides information on diet, nutrition and related health matters, and organizes scientific conferences and seminars; in addition, a range of scientific publications is produced, along with a regular newsletter, and resources for teachers.

Cancer Research UK
Angel Building
407 St John Street
London EC1V 4AD
Tel.: 020 7242 0200 (Switchboard); 0300 123 1022 (Supporter services)
Website: www.cancerresearchuk.org

The Healthy Living section of the website provides nutritional information.

Memorial Sloan-Kettering Cancer Center
1275 York Avenue
New York, NY 10065
Website: www.mskcc.org

The Memorial Sloan-Kettering Cancer Center provides an excellent online nutrition search resource which provides an overview of the evidence for nutrition supplement and herb products.

Patients on Intravenous and Nasogastric Nutrition Therapy (PINNT)
PO Box 3126
Christchurch
Dorset BH23 2XS
Tel.: 01202 481625
Website: www.pinnt.com

Founded to help people who require intravenous or nasogastric feeding, and their families.

Penny Brohn Cancer Care
Chapel Pill Lane
Pill
Bristol BS20 0HH
Tel.: 01275 370100 (general); 0845 123 2310 (helpline)
Website: www.pennybrohncancercare.org

Offers a holistic approach to people with cancer. Nutritional help is provided on the website under the Our Therapies section.

World Cancer Research Fund (WCRF UK)
22 Bedford Square
LondonWC1B 3HH
Tel.: 020 7343 4205
Website: www.wcrf-uk.org

A charity dedicated to research around lifestyle and prevention of cancer. There are lots of great nutritional resources which can be ordered or downloaded from the cancer prevention section of the website.

General

Macmillan Cancer Support
89 Albert Embankment
London SE1 7UQ
Tel.: 020 7840 7840; information line: 0808 808 0000 (9 a.m. to 8 p.m., Monday to Friday)
Website: www.macmillan.org.uk

Marie Curie Cancer Care
Supporter Services Team
89 Albert Embankment
London SE1 7TP
Tel.: 020 7599 7777 (general); 0800 716 146 (free helpline, 9 a.m. to 5.30 p.m., Monday to Friday)
Website: www.mariecurie.org.uk

This organization provides free end-of-life care to those who are terminally ill, either at home or in one of their nine hospices. There are also head offices in Northern Ireland. Scotland and Wales (see below), all sharing the same website.

Marie Curie Cancer Care (Northern Ireland)
1a Kensington Road
Belfast BT5 6NF
Tel.: 028 9088 2032

Marie Curie Cancer Care (Scotland)
14 Links Place
Edinburgh EH6 3EB
Tel.: 0131 561 3900

Marie Curie Cancer Care (Wales)
Mamhilad House
Mamhilad Park Estate
Pontypool NP4 0HZ
Tel.: 01495 740818

Nutrition products

Abbott Nutrition
Abbott House
Vanwall Business Park
Vanwall Road
Maidenhead
Berkshire SL6 4XE
Tel.: 01628 773355 (Switchboard); 0800 252 882 (Freephone Nutrition Helpline)
Website: www.abbottnutrition.co.uk

Supplies a wide variety of nutritional products and services, including the Ensure Plus range, to help people at risk of malnutrition because of eating difficulties. The website contains recipes.

Nutricia Ltd
White Horse Business Park
Newmarket Avenue
Trowbridge
Wiltshire BA14 0XQ
Tel.: 01225 711677
Website: www.nutricia.co.uk

This range of nutritional solutions is for use solely under the supervision of healthcare professionals.

Further reading

Bor, Professor Robert, Dr Carina Eriksen and Ceilidh Stapelkamp, *Coping with the Psychological Effects of Cancer*, London, Sheldon Press, 2010.

Harvie, Dr Michelle and Roy Ackermann, *The Genesis Breast Cancer Prevention Diet*, New York, Rodale, 2006.

McVicar, Jekka, *Jekka's Complete Herb Book*, London, Kyle Cathie, 2009.

Priestman, Dr Terry, *Coping with Breast Cancer*, London, Sheldon Press, 2006.

Priestman, Dr Terry, *Coping with Radiotherapy*, London, Sheldon Press, 2007.

Priestman, Dr Terry, *Reducing Your Risk of Cancer*, London, Sheldon Press, 2008.

Priestman, Dr Terry, *Coping with Chemotherapy*, new edition, London, Sheldon Press, 2009.

Priestman, Dr Terry, *The Cancer Survivor's Handbook*, London, Sheldon Press, 2009.

Shaw, Dr Clare and the Royal Marsden Hospital, *Cancer: Food, Facts and Recipes. The Power of Food – Food, Facts and Recipes*, London, Hamlyn, 2005.

Shaw, Dr Clare, *Nutrition and Cancer*, London, Wiley-Blackwell, 2010.

Index

NB: Recipes are entered in *italics*.

acid reflux 90
active stage, treatment 2
activity
    lack of 123
    see also exercise
acupuncture 76
advanced cancers 29
Agricultural Research Service (USA) 64
alcohol 7, 16, 95, 123, 128
    drinking guidelines 116, 128
alcohol-based disinfectants 119
alkylresorcinols 64, 65
almond milk 109
alternative medicine 122
American Institute for Cancer Research
    (AICR) 15, 134–5
amino acids 48, 125
anaemia 36, 93
anise 69
anorexia 22
antacid medication 92
anti-diarrhoea medications 94
anti-emetic pills 76
antioxidants 55–6, 136
    ORAC capacity 64, 65
    wholegrains 64–5
    see also polyphenols
appetite 1
    alcohol 128
    decreased 30–1
    food tips 102–3
    increased 24
    loss 22, 102–3, 130–1
    monitoring 27
    weight changes 74
aromatherapy 76
ascites 31
avenanthramides 64
avoiding foods 98, 120, 124

basil 69
basil soup, roasted tomato and 82–3
beef 63, 129
beef stroganoff, easy 88
berries, dark 138
berry smoothie 108
best practice 12

betaine 65
beverages *see* drinks
Bimuno® 95
biological therapies 42
biscuits, high protein muesli 59
bitter taste 82
black pepper 69
bloating 52, 97
blood
    blood cells 19–20
    blood count 19–20
    blood pressure 92, 93
    blood sugar levels 93, 126, 127
    chemotherapy impact 36–7
blueberry and banana muffin 47
body
    key functions 43
    weight *see* weight
body, cancer/treatment impact 18–19
    cachexia 22–4
    normal functions 19–22
body mass index (BMI) 31–2, 33
bolus feeding 75
bone marrow 19, 35
bovine growth hormones 125
bowel 19
    cancers 94
    enteral feeding 113
    function 52
    large 94
    problems 37, 73
    radiotherapy 40
    small 90, 94
    surgery 94, 95
brain 21
    cancer 29, 40
    glucose/sugar 126
bran muffin 46–7
bread 63–5, 99, 137
breakfast 50, 78, 100, 138
breast cancer 26, 29, 40, 125, 129, 130
the brew 101, 109
Build-up drinks 111, 147
build-up trolley vs weight-management
    trolley 115–17
bulk recipes 86
butter vs margarine 61

cachexia 22–4, 35, 127
  symptoms 23
calcium 58, 90, 93, 125
Caloreen energy powder 112, 147
calories 9, 24, 105, 130, 132
  high-calorie drinks *see* nutrition sip
    drinks
Calshake powder 109, 111, 148
cancer
  advanced 29
  -associated nutritional problems
    28–30
  causes 5
cancer prevention 133–45
  cooking, enjoyment/health 139–41
  diet 134–5
  superfoods 135–6
  WCRF guidelines 129, 133–4
cancer/treatment, impact 2–3, 15–26
  key stages 15–18
cans, hygiene 118
capsaicin 136
carbohydrates 22, 23, 93, 99, 126–7
  slow vs fast release 44–5, 45–6
  supplements 105
carcinogens 129
carotenoids 55, 64
cashew milk 109
celebration, eating as 139–41, 143–4
cell repair 20
cereals 96, 99, 116
cervix, radiotherapy 40
chai tea 83–4
cheese 99, 126
chemicals 135, 136
chemoradiation 39
chemotherapy 9, 24, 35–9
  blood, impact 36–7
  preparation 37–9
  side effects 36–7
chicken curry 68–9
chicken pasta, easy creamy 87–8
chicken soup 79–80
chocolate coffee shake 80
chocolate, dark 135
choline 65
chopping boards, hygiene 118
cinnamic acid 136
cloves 70
coffee 95
coffee shake, chocolate 80
cold foods 82, 95
colorectal cancer 129
common questions 124–32
Complan drinks 111, 149

complementary medicine 122
'complete feeds' 104
'complete source of nutrition' 104
condiments 116
conjugated linolenic acids 125
constipation 52, 96–7
  food tips 96–7
contraceptive pills 125
cooking 119
  enjoyment/health 139–41
  programme, school 143
  utensils, hygiene 118
corn jacket potatoes, tuna and 66
cottage cheese 126
cramps, late dumping syndrome 93
cream 99
curcumin 68

daily energy/nutrient allowance 43–7
daily record, food intake 2, 130, 132
dairy foods 19, 48, 99, 115
  avoiding 124–6
defrosting food 120
dehydration 53, 54, 94
Department of Agriculture (USA) 65
depression 93
desserts 101
  ready-to-drink 110–12
diarrhoea 54, 93, 94–6, 124
  food tips 94–5
diary, food 2, 130, 132
dietary fibres 65
dietitians, role 11–14
diets 5, 7–9
  alternative 122–3
  cancer prevention 134–5
  changes 3
  following treatment 26
  guidelines 11, 132
  influences 10
  soft/purée 97–101
  special *see* special diets
digestive system
  cachexia 23
  digestive tract 19, 36
  enzymes 90
dinner (main meals) 78, 100, 139
Dioralyte 95
disease-related malnutrition 9
dishwasher, hygiene 118
disinfectants 119
distraction, therapy 76
drinks 82, 101, 107, 138
  recipes 108–9
  see also nutrition sip drinks

drip feeding 75
dumping syndrome 92–3, 94

early dumping syndrome 92
easy beef stroganoff 88
easy creamy chicken pasta 87–8
eating well 43–71
    action-packed treatment foods
        56–65
    daily energy/nutrient allowances
        43–7
    Eatwell Plates 56, 57, 58
    fats 50–2
    fibre 52–3
    fruit/vegetable nutrients 71
    protein 47–50
    recipes 65–71
    vitamins/minerals 54–6
    water 53–4
    see also nutrition
*Eating Well and Being Active Following
    Cancer Treatment* (Freeman) 18, 26,
    134
Eatwell Plates 56
    build-up 58
    high protein 57
education, continuing 12
eggs 98, 119
    allowance 59–61
    recipes 60–1
eicosapentaenoic acid (EPA) 52
endocrine issues 25
endometrial cancers 29
energy 12, 17, 21, 43–7
    -dense foods 16
    high energy drinks 108, 111
    immune system 19–20, 21
    powders 111–12
Enshake powder 109, 111
Ensure Plus drink 37, 146
enteral feeding 75, 113, 114
environmental exposure 7
enzymes 55, 90
equipment 117
Escherichia coli 120
exercise 24, 97, 132
    benefits 25–6
expertise, nutrition 13

fast release carbohydrates 126–7
fatigue 24, 54, 85–8
    food tips 85–7
    recipes 87–8
fats 22, 23, 31, 105, 116
    avoiding 129–30

eating well 50–2
    types 51
fatty foods 94
feeling full 91–2
fennel 70
ferulic acid 64
fibre 44, 52–3, 94
    -enriched products 110
fish 52, 62, 98
fish cakes 62–3
flavonoids 64
flavour 81, 116
    mixes 82–5
flaxseed mighty mix 62
flaxseeds 61–2, 96
fluid 54, 94, 97
    build-up 31
    see also water
FODMAP foods 16, 53
food
    diary 2, 130, 132
    memories 142–3
    presentation 131
    range 131
    storage 119
Food Fix suggestions (author's) 37, 52, 72,
        81, 106
*Food, Nutrition, Physical Activity, and
    the Prevention of Cancer: a global
    perspective* (WCRF/AICR 2007)
    134
food safety 118–23
    alternative diets 122–3
    food hygiene 38, 118–20
    food poisoning 120–1
    foods to avoid 120
    vitamins/minerals 121–2
food supplements 146–9
    cautions 16, 36, 54–5
    costs 13, 123
    prescribed 92
    safety 121–2
    see also nutrition sip drinks
Fortisip sip feed drink 37, 147
Fresubin Energy Drink range 148
fromage frais 99
fruit 16, 26, 99, 115
    -based drink/meal supplements 110
    boosting intake 67
    carbohydrates 44
    constipation 97
    dark coloured 66–8
    juicing 130
    nutrients, retaining 71
    polyphenols 137–8

washing 118, 129
fruit salad smoothie 108
fruity protein shake 80
full-fat milk 56
functional gastrointestinal symptoms 53

garlic 70
gastrointestinal tract 40
    cancers 90–1
genetics 7
ginger squash, refreshing 79–80
glucose 21, 93, 126–7
Glycaemic Index (GI) 44, 46–7, 126–7,
    132
Glycaemic Load (GL) 44
gogi berry 135
grain foods 116
group sessions, nutrition 142
guacamole 84
gut immunity 19
gynaecological cancers 29

hair 35
    follicles 19
    loss 25
hand hygiene 118, 119
head, cancers 28, 40
health benefits, nutrition 144
Health and Care Professions Council
    (HCPC) 13
heart 21, 50
    disease 23
herbs 68–71, 116, 137
    remedies 122
high calorie products 103, 110
    drinks *see* nutrition sip drinks
high GI type carbohydrates 126–7
high protein fruity shakes 59
high protein muesli biscuits 59
higher-fibre foods 19
high-fibre food 94
HIV (human immunodeficiency virus)
    23
hormonal cancer 124–6
hormonal therapies 24, 41–2
hormone sources 125
hot foods 82, 95
hunger 132
hydration 132
hygiene, food 38, 118–20
    handling food 119–20
    tips 118–19
hyponatremia 53

iced coffee 109

immune system 19–20, 21
Imodium 94
indigestion 92
individual, tailored approach 12, 13–14
infection 10, 12
    immunity 20
    preventing *see* food safety
insoluble fibre 52
insulin 93, 127
    resistance 25
intensive farming methods 125
internet 13
Ipee Daily (iPhone app) 54
iron 36, 63, 90, 92
irritable bowel syndrome (IBS) 95

Journal of Clinical Oncology 122
juice 99
    juicing fruit/vegetables 130

kidneys 21, 23

lactose 19, 126
lactose-free milk 58, 126
lamb 63, 129
late dumping syndrome 93
laxatives 97
leftovers 120
lemon curd 60–1
lethargy 24
lifestyle 15, 125
liquid supplements *see* nutrition sip
    drinks
listeria 120
liver 21
Living Well programme 13
low FODMAP diet 95
low GI type carbohydrates 126–7
low GI type cereals 132
lower gastrointestinal tract, nutritional risk
    and cancer of 29
low-fat dairy foods 125
luecine 125
lunch 78, 138–9
lung cancer 23, 29, 40, 129
lungs 21
lycopene 55

mackerel 62
macronutrient allowances 44
main meals (dinners) 78, 100, 139
major organs 21
malnourishment, overweight 27–8
malnutrition, disease-related 9
Malnutrition Screening Tool (MST) 30

margarine vs butter 61
Maxi Joule powder and liquid 149
Maxijul energy powder 112, 147
MaxPro powders/gels 112, 149
Max-Sorb gel 149
meat 63, 98, 119
  processed 129
  raw 120
  red 16, 48, 129
medications
  concerns 73
  unhelpful 38
menopause, earlier onset 24
metallic taste 82
metastatic cancers 29
Mexican flavour mix 84–5
milk 99, 125
  allowance 56, 58–9
  -based supplements 110
  lactose-free 58, 126
milkshakes 80, 111
minerals 44, 111
  eating well 54–6
  food safety 121–2
mint 70
monitoring nutrition 27–33
mono-unsaturated fats 51
mood swings 93
mouth 36, 82, 124
muesli biscuits, high protein 59
muffins
  blueberry and banana muffin 47
  bran muffin 46–7
muscle changes 31
  loss 11, 21
music, therapy 76

nasoduodenal feeding 113
nasogastric feeding 113
nasojejunal feeding 113
nausea and vomiting 37, 75–85, 124
  daily food schedule 78
  food tips 76–8
  recipes 79–80
neck cancers 28, 40
neurological tumours 29
neutropenia 36–7
new start, key stage 4 18
NHS (National Health Service) 12
nibbles 22, 76
  see also snacks
nil by mouth 89
nitrates 128
normal functions 19–22
nut-flavoured smoothie drink 109

nutrients 7
  daily allowance 43–7
  fruit/vegetable, retaining 71
nutrition
  in cancer 7–14
  changes 11
  engaging with 2–4
  following treatment 26
  group sessions 142
  guidelines 123
  monitoring 27–33
  problems, cancer-associated 28–30
  treatment effects 34–5, 35–42
  treatment support 9–10
  see also cooking; eating well
nutrition sip drinks 17, 37, 103, 104–12,
    146–9
  home-made 108–9
  points to consider 105–7
  prescribable 12
  range 107–8
  ready-to-drink products 110–12
  using 104–5
'nutritionally complete' products
    110–11
nuts 137

obesity 32, 129
oedema 31
oesophagus 40, 91
oils 50–1, 61, 116
  fish 52, 62
  polyphenols 138
olives 137
omega 3 fatty acids 50, 61
ORAC (oxygen radical absorbance capacity)
    score 64, 65
organic foods 128–9
oryzonol 64
osteoporosis 125
ovaries 40
over-hydration 53
overweight, malnourishment 27–8

palate
  clearing 82
  of colour 144
palliative care, key stage 3 18
pancakes, protein 50
pancreas 40, 90, 91
parenteral nutrition 75, 113, 114
pelvic region 40
percentage weight loss 32
percutaneous endoscopic gastrostomy
    (PEG) 113

personalized food plan 12
pets, hygiene 118
pharmaceutical drug approval 121
Phenol Explorer database 135, 136
phenolic lipids 64
phenolics 64, 136
physical activity 16
phytates 64
phytochemicals 55–6, 135
phytonutrients 44, 55–6, 139, 140
phyto-oestrogen supplements 130
phytosterols 55, 64
pick-your-own fields 143
pitta bread 63–5
plain yoghurt lassi 109
plant foods 16, 52, 123
    polyphenols 135–8
platin-based chemotherapy 52
poisoning, food 120–1
Polycal energy powder 112, 147
Polycose energy powder 112, 146
polyphenols 64, 136–7
    plant foods 135–8
    top 100 137
polyunsaturated fats 51
popcorn snack 65–6
pork 129
potassium 63
potatoes 63–5, 99
potatoes, tuna and corn jacket 66
poultry 98
pre-biotics 95
prevention, key stage 1 15–17
priorities, good nutrition 6
Pro-Cal shots 112, 148
processed meat 129
Prosource 112, 149
prostate cancer 29, 40
protein
    distribution 50
    eating well 47–50
    extra amounts 76, 132
    foods providing 48, 49, 58, 98,
        115
    gels/liquids 112
    guidelines 48–9
    high biological value 48
    powders 108, 111–12
    recipes 50, 59
    requirements 9, 21, 22, 23
    supplements 105
protein pancakes 50
Protifar powders/gels 112, 147
psychological impact 21
pulses 98

puréed foods
    balance 98, 100
    diet 97, 101
    preparation 97

quasi-nutritionists 13, 56
questions, common 124–32
Quorn 98

radiologically inserted gastrostomy feeding
        (RIG) 113
radiotherapy (radiation therapy) 39–40
    preparation 39–40
    side effects 39, 40
raw food 119, 120
ready-to-drink products 110–12
readymade meals 86
recipes 65–71
    adapting 140–1
    high protein 59, 60, 80
    home-made nutrition sip drinks
        108–9
    nausea and vomiting 79–80
    rehydration 95–6
    slow/fast release carbohydrates 46
    soft textures 101
    taste changes 82–5
recovery, treatment 20
rectum 40
red blood cells 19–20, 36
red meats 16, 48, 129
red wine 135
redcurrants 137
reflux 90, 92
refreshing ginger squash 79–80
refrigerator, hygiene 119–20
rehydration 94, 95
relaxation, therapy 76
Resource drink 37, 147
resveratrol 55, 136
rice 63–5
rich foods 19
risks, nutrition and cancer types 28
roasted tomato and basil soup 82–3
rosemary 70
rosmarinic acid 136

safety *see* food safety
St Mark's oral rehydration solution 95–6
salmon 62
salmonella 120
salt intake 16
sardines 62
saturated fats 51
Scandishake powder 111, 147

scientific literature 12
scrambled eggs 60
screening, nutritional problems, risks
    30–1
Sea-Band 78
seeds 137
selenium 55, 65
semi-skimmed milk 56
sesame oil 61
shopping, planning 43
side effects 3, 72–88, 127
    fatigue 85–8
    food combating 72–5
    nausea and vomiting 75–85
    support feeding 112–17
    taste changes 81–5
    see also constipation; diarrhoea;
        surgery
sip feed drinks *see* nutrition sip drinks
skimmed milk powder 56, 58–9
skin 35
slow cookers 88
slow-release carbohydrates 126–7
small amounts, weight management
    132
small bowel 90
smoking 123, 134
snacks 78, 131
    superfood suggestions 139
social eating 4, 6, 18
    celebration 139–41, 143–4
soft textures 97–101
    diet 97
    tips 98–9
soluble fibre 52
soup bases 109
soups 111
    ready-to-drink 110–12
soy sauce 73
soya foods 98, 130
special diets 39
    drinks 123
    feeds 12
specialist team 27
sphincter (stomach) 90
sphingolipids 64
spices 68–71, 116, 137
spinal cord 40
sports market 38, 105, 108
stamina 3, 21
steroids 24
stomach
    cancer 40, 93
    role of 90–1
    surgery 91–2, 92–3

stomach soother 80
storage, food 119
strength 3
    muscle loss 21
strong flavours 81
sugar
    avoiding 126–7
    cravings 25
    sugary foods 24
super-green smoothie 109
superfoods
    cancer prevention 135–9
    suggestions 138–9
supplements *see* food supplements;
        nutrition sip drinks
support feeding 112–17
    at home 114
    build-up trolley vs weight-management
        trolley 115–17
    stocking up 114
surgery 40–1, 89–90
    bowel 94, 95
    impact 112
    preparation 41
    side effects 40–1
    stomach 91–2, 92–3, 94
swallowing passage 93
sweet dishes *see* desserts
sweet taste 82

tailored approach 12, 13–14
taste
    bitter 82
    metallic 82
    nutrition and 144
    sense of 73
    sweet 82
taste changes 81–5
    food tips 81–2
    recipes 82–5
tea 95, 137
tea, chai 83–4
temperature, nutrition and 144
textures 81, 144
    see also soft textures
thymol 136
tinned food 86
tobacco 134
tocopherols 64
tocotrienols 64
tofu 98
tomato and basil soup, roasted 82–3
trans-fatty acids 51
treatment 34–42
    action-packed foods 56–65

active stage 2
combinations 7–8, 18, 39
impact *see* cancer/treatment, impact
key stage 2 17
nutrition, effects 34–5, 35–42
nutrition following 26
outcomes 10
recovery 20
side effects 3, 34, 38, 127
support 9–10
types 35
treats 38–9, 117, 132
tumours 90, 112, 130
tuna 62
tuna and corn jacket potatoes 66
turmeric 68, 135

umami 144
upper gastrointestinal tract 28
urine 54
uterus 40

vagus nerve 91, 94
vegetables 16, 26, 99, 115
　boosting intake 67–8
　carbohydrates 44
　constipation 97
　dark coloured 66–8
　extra 132
　juicing 130
　nutrients, retaining 71
　polyphenols 137–8
　soft textures 100
　washing 118, 129
　weight management 132
Vitajoule energy powder 112, 148
vital organs 21
vitamin A 55
vitamin B 63
vitamin B12 63, 90, 92, 93
vitamin C 55, 128
vitamin E 55, 64
vitamins 44
　eating well 54–6
　food safety 121–2
　supplement drinks 111

Vitapro 112, 148
vomiting *see* nausea and vomiting

washing
　fruit/vegetables 118, 129
　hands 118, 119
wasting syndrome *see* cachexia
water
　filter, hygiene 118–19
　importance 53–4
　intake 38
　recommendations 53–4
weight
　changes 13, 21–2, 27, 28
　gain 24–5, 131–2
　stability 5, 16
weight loss 8, 29, 130–1
　percentage 32
　screening 30–1
　see also cachexia
weight-management tips 132
weight-management trolley vs build-up
　　trolley 115–17
whey protein 126
white blood cells 19–20, 36–7
whole milk 56, 99
wholegrains 26, 63–4, 96
　antioxidants 64–5
　carbohydrates 44
　quantity 132
wholemeal 63–4
wind 52, 92, 97
wine, red 135
'wonder diets' 123
work surfaces, hygiene 118
World Cancer Research Fund (WCRF) 16,
　　26
　2007 Expert Report (with AICR) 15–16,
　　134
　cancer prevention guidelines 129,
　　133–4

yoghurt 99

zinc 55, 63, 81